Krishna Warrior Fitness Challenge

The Workout of Your Life

By Arkadiusz Madej

First printing 2010

Interior design and layout by BookMasters, Inc.

Cover art and design by Greg Madej/Steel Soul Productions www.gregsartdomain.com

Photos by Richard New/www.PureNewVision.com

Printed in the United States of America

ISBN: 978-0-9769507-3-8

Persons interested in the subject matter are invited to visit publisher's Web site:

www.krishnawarriors.com

DISCLAIMER:
The author of this material is not responsible in any manner whatsoever for any injury that may occur through following the instructions contained in this material. The activities, physical and otherwise, described herein for informational purposes only, may be too strenuous for some people, and the reader should consult a physician before engaging in them. Before practicing the exercises in this book, be sure that your equipment is in good condition and do not take risks beyond your level of training and fitness. Furthermore, the exercise programs and nutritional recommendations in this book are not intended as a substitute for any exercise routine or dietary regimen that may have been prescribed by your doctor. If you have a health problem, before you embark on any fitness or nutritional program, seek clearance from a qualified physician.

WORKS BY ARKADIUSZ MADEJ

Transcendental Warrior I
Serving in the Army of Lord Krishna

Transcendental Warrior II
Let the Battle Begin

Transcendental Warrior III
Clearing the Battlefield

Krishna Warrior Fitness Challenge
The Workout of Your Life

DEDICATION

"Whatever you do, whatever you eat, whatever you offer or give away, and whatever austerities you perform—do that, O warrior, as an offering to Me (Krishna)."

(Bhagavad-Gita 9.27)

With dedication to my eternal master, Srila Prabhupada, who is always fearless at the feet of the Lord, and at whose feet all masters sit.

A real treasure to own. Delivers a down-to-earth vision on exercise, body training, and health. It will guide you to a healthier body and newfound energy. This is a must-read.

Kathy Boand, Arizona

FOREWORD

There are many books on exercise, meditation, and health that treat each in detail from the author's point of view. These are all very helpful in their own way. As a martial artist searching for the path to expand his own boundaries, these books always struggle with the way to make their path yours, give an incomplete picture on how to accomplish your goals, and if one is successful it is usually brief. In essence they provide an incomplete picture of an incomplete path. A holistic point of view is needed to show one a path to continually expand his or her boundaries. It needs to address the strengths and weaknesses of one's mind, body, and their journey together since they are not separate. Ark provides such a path in great detail in this book.

For me as a martial artist, the focus of my fitness training has been on combat-oriented movements with weights, which has resulted in sharpened techniques, increased speed, more energy, and increased sensitivity. The increased stamina has allowed me to expand my exercise routine in all areas. I noticed some immediate changes in my body and mind. The most enjoyable aspect of my training is the variety and difficulty of exercises, which concentrate on my weaknesses.

The attention to the proper form of each exercise was a significant factor in my improvement but an exercise is not useful without the mindfulness to push one to accomplish it. The benefits of increased health are incomplete without the enjoyment of accomplishing physically and mentally challenging activities. The mind cannot be sharpened without the body taking part. These are the tools that Ark provides to be a warrior in all aspects of the word.

James Anthony Sublett
Rank: 3rd Dan, World Tae Kwon Do Federation
Kaya Martial Arts, Arlington Heights, IL
Master Sung Min Park 7th Dan, World Tae Kwon Do Federation

ACKNOWLEDGMENTS

I would like to thank Xsport Fitness team for allowing me to use their facility to take most of the photos used in this book. Thank you, Danny. Thank you Steve, Uncle Damon, Mel, my general manager, and all others too numerous to mention. Thank you for your ongoing support. It's been great training, guys …

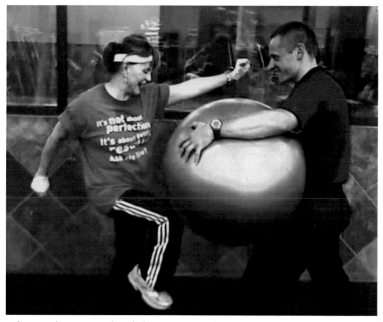

Client Blanca and Ark have trained together for 5 years and still meet three times a week for the workout of their lives!

I would like to thank the Oak Brook Park District for allowing me to film the video in their facility.

I want to also send a deep thank you to my karate instructor, Shihan Leslaw Samitowski, for setting the foundation of my fitness, without which I would not be the same kind of trainer I am today.

Furthermore, I would like to thank my dear brother, Greg Madej, for creating, among many other things in this project, the front and back cover page of the *Krishna Warrior Fitness Challenge*. I would like to thank Rich New for his great effort in taking the photos for the Krishna Warrior book and Krzys Skinderowicz for polishing them. I would like to thank

Bill Yauch for making the demo DVD of the *Krishna Warrior Fitness Challenge*. I would like to thank Kim D. and Susan H. for participating in the video and posing for pictures in the book. I would also like to thank Kim G., Bill H., and Marcin L. for posing for pictures in the book. I would like to give special thanks to Ragavardhan Das for allowing me to use his music from *Transcendental Village* in my demo DVD. I would like to thank Kasia for spending many hours to compile a concise index.

I would like to thank all of my clients who have trained with me over the years, and especially those who have written testimonials used in this book. I would like to thank my friend Brian Mueller for being the first person to purchase my *Transcendental Warrior* book before it even came out. I thank you for your wonderful new member tours at Xsport as well.

And last but not least, I thank warriors Jerry, Todd, Revo, and Ed for hailing the transcendental vibrations of Hare Krishna throughout the gym. *Haaaree Krishnaaa! Krishna Warriors! Krishna Warriors!* I would like to thank warrior Chadd who melodiously sings Hare Krishna, and my former fitness manager, Tyler, for amplifying the vibration, and all the other warriors who join in.

TABLE OF CONTENTS

INVOKING AUSPICIOUSNESS

I was born in the darkest ignorance, and my spiritual master opened my eyes with the torch of knowledge. Let me offer my respectful obeisance unto him. Let me offer my respectful obeisance to my spiritual master, by whose inspiration I have been engaged in many battles for the Lord.

Let me also offer my humble obeisance to all of Krishna's warriors who have come in my spiritual master's line.

My dear Lord Krishna, You are the greatest warrior of all. Your all-attractive form subdues every living entity's heart by its sublime beauty. You are the ultimate protector of every devotee at all times. Indeed, You are the shelter of us all. Let me offer my respectful obeisance unto Your lotus feet.

Let me offer my humble obeisance unto the lotus feet of Their Lordships Sri Sri Kishore Kishori of Chicago, by whose mercy this unqualified person attempts to spread the science of Krishna warriors to the modern world of fitness.

INTRODUCTION

ANOTHER FITNESS BOOK?

Just how many fitness books have you read or browsed through? Dozens? Hundreds, right? And you, fitness experts? I bet you looked through thousands of those books and articles, haven't you? So why are fitness books still being written? Because we are discovering new needs for different fitness enthusiasts, and we are learning more about our bodies every day. We are putting old and new together in different formats to address different needs that you, fitness enthusiasts, might have. That is why new books and articles are still being written, and that is why fitness bibles are often corrected and brought up to date.

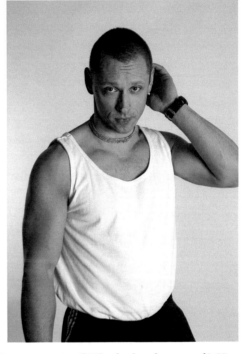

So what can you find in this book that you won't find in any other book that's on the shelf out there? You will find a genuine way of how to transform your body, mind, and rediscover your real spirit as a warrior of Krishna. Did I hear you say, "What's that last word? You said 'Kreeshna'?" Some of you fitness experts may not be finding "Krishna" in your fitness dictionary.

Yes, "Krishna." Krishna is a word for God that historically derives from India. The old historical accounts tell us that Krishna was here on earth some 5,000 years ago. Not only was He a superb warrior, but He also disseminated knowledge to other warriors on how to develop their minds to the highest potential. So since I have always wanted to be a warrior and have studied Krishna science for years, I felt inspired to introduce Krishna to the world of holistic fitness.

Let me tell you, it is a lot of fun to be a Krishna warrior. If you have a problem with this foreign-sounding word, you can use your own word for God. Oh, by the way, in the *Krishna Warrior Fitness Challenge*, you can expect to find various never-before-practiced-or-seen-by-you exercises that Krishna warriors use.

WHO IS THIS BOOK FOR?

If you ever desired to be healthy on all three levels—that is, body, mind, and spirit—this book is for you. If you ever wanted to learn uncommon exercises that you don't usually learn from even fitness trainers, this book is for you. If you ever wanted to call yourself a warrior, this book will make you a real warrior. If you ever wanted to exercise for health and fitness and not for competition, this book is for you. If you were never really good at any sport but deep inside you wanted to be the best at something, this book will make you reach for the best within yourself and bring you the true medal of achievement. If you always avoided exercise because you had no plan or motivation, this book gives a definite plan of action surcharged with spiritual motivation. If you ever wanted to achieve functional strength for daily life, this book is for you. If you ever wanted to be as fit as some of the best martial artists, this book will accomplish that. If you ever wanted to have fun with your exercise routine, this book will not bore you.

As a fitness book, it will walk you through uncommon workouts designed to develop functional strength for life. Designed for fit beginners, intermediate, and advanced fitness enthusiasts, it is recommended especially for them. However, even athletes who practice specific disciplines might find something for themselves. In *Krishna Warrior Fitness Challenge,* you will find various ways to enhance your mind and spirit for the purpose of your own sport or activity.

So what are you waiting for, warrior? Go to the next page and *get ready* for the workout of your life!

BASIC PRINCIPLES

THREEFOLD BODIES

There are some important things to understand about fitness that I think you ought to know. First of all, we as Krishna warriors work on three levels: body, mind, and soul (spirit). Therefore, every one of our workouts will have three dimensions. This is holistic fitness.

As human beings, we work by summoning three tools: our will, our attention, and our body. If you don't want to do something, but you are forced to do it, you will not enjoy it. Furthermore, you will pay less attention to what you are doing. Without the power of your will and applying your attention to what you do, your work will have little value; it will not bring the best results. That is why we will start every workout with meditation, then we will proceed to work out, and we will finish the workout with meditation.

The underlying principle of any kind of work is subtle energy of mind and intelligence. When you develop faith in what you are doing and the goal that lies ahead, you will actually manifest its reality in the physical realm. For example, if I want to have a new body, I first decide what kind of body I want. Then I decide what my present body will need as far as nutrition and training to transform itself into a higher-class machine.

Your body is a machine. Just take a chariot as an example. You are the passenger in the chariot, the mind is the reins, the intelligence is the driver, and the horses are your senses (eyes for seeing, nose for smelling, legs for locomotion, etc.). Therefore, to perfectly achieve our goal, we must know how to drive the chariot of our body safely and properly.

In our workout chapters, which start with the beginner Krishna warrior program, we will always begin with the Castle of Intelligence and the Castle of Mind. These first portions educate the trainee about the subtle energies involved in improving one's character and building discipline, which, in turn, will affect the workout itself. Then we will proceed to exercises.

THE QUALIFYING ENTRANCE POINT

Get on the floor and crank out at least 30 push-ups in good form (arms half bent)—that is, if you are a warrior in a man's body. For warriors in female bodies, you need at least 15 push-ups without the use of knees. Next, do 50 sit-ups in good form (halfway up, keeping hands up and crossed on your chest). As for you ladies, you can give me 30. If you can't do that, I recommend that you start a more basic training program, continue it for a few months, and that will get you to a fit beginner level. Only then, using the *Krishna Warrior Fitness Challenge* (KWFC) book will prove effective and rewarding. In other words, you need to be in at least an average shape to undertake the Krishna Warrior Challenge.

PERIODIZATION PRINCIPLE

Periodization is based on the premise that training methods can be arranged in a way that each training period, or phase, benefits from the period before it (Staley 9). When the training program is not periodized, it lacks variation of exercise intensity, volume, or content, and its results are much less predictable. Those who do not implement periodization into their training program usually stay in relatively the same shape, and changes in their physical condition are rather unexpected (10).

The concept of periodization has been practiced and tested for many years by Russian athletes. It is by far the best way to maximize the effectiveness of your workouts and minimize the risks of overtraining because it alternates easy, moderate, and intense training sessions (2 Hatfield 421). For example, as a beginner who is in average shape, you can start with the strength training plan three times a week that is contained in this book. On the other 3 days, you either jog, ride a bike, play your favorite sport, or do skill training (sparring, other technical drills specific to your sport) for 30 minutes to an hour. Take 1 complete rest day where you do not engage in any physical activity. Remember the saying, "The best athletes are those who know how to relax between efforts."

As an aspiring Krishna warrior, your training cycle will be divided into different training cycles: macrocycles, mesoscycles, and microcycles. A macrocycle refers to the entire training period, by the end of which, you should reach your goal (e.g., losing 20 pounds of fat, putting on 10 pounds of muscle, or just becoming stronger). The *Krishna Warrior Fitness Challenge* book contains one macrocycle. It should take you at least 18 weeks to complete the training programs in the book.

A mesocycle is a division within a macrocycle. For example, in the KWFC book, you will have three different workout plans: beginner, intermediate, and advanced. Each program should be practiced for at least 6 weeks before you move on to the next level. It could be that you are able to perform each exercise correctly in a certain workout plan, but you still take too long of a rest between exercises or sequences. Thus, you should work on endurance and improve your time. (Or, as an option, you could use progressions featured at the end of each exercise to go to the next level of difficulty and continue for another couple of weeks.) Keep in mind that the workouts featured here are NONSTOP ones.

A microcycle is a division within a mesocycle. One week of following the training program would count as a microcycle. For example, Monday, Wednesday, and Friday would be your Krishna Warrior Fitness Challenge days. Then Tuesday, Thursday, and Saturday would be your "easy workout" days or sports-specific training days. After completing 6 of such weeks, you will have completed one mesocycle. A microcycle can be further divided into training sessions which have three basic components: meditation and warm-up; the exercises, cooldown, and stretching; and finally, meditation.

THE SAID PRINCIPLE

The Specific Adaptation to Imposed Demands (SAID) principle is one of the seven grand-daddy laws of strength training. It states that if your training objective is to become more explosive, then you must train explosively. If you would like cardiovascular benefit, then you must tax the heart muscle along with other muscles without taking long breaks between exercises. In the Krishna Warrior Challenge program, you will learn from the description of the exercises presented that many of them help in increasing the power of kicks and punches (as in karate, for example). As my background is in martial arts, I attempted to develop and present many exercises that are specific to either karate or core strengthening (as core is the foundation of your body's physical movements in all sports). So although each workout plan (beginner, intermediate, and advanced) develops your whole body, it puts emphasis on abdominal and lower back areas (commonly known as "core") and karate-specific exercises.

PERIPHERAL HEART ACTION

The framework for the Krishna Warrior Fitness Challenge program is based on Peripheral Heart Action (PHA), a system developed by Dr. Arthur Steinhaus in the 1960s. PHA was later popularized by former Mr. America and Mr. Universe, Bob Gajda.

Peripheral Heart Action is a cardio form of training that adds resistance and is conducted in a circuitlike fashion. It has been used by many athletes to burn fat without losing muscle. John McCallum, author of *The Complete Keys to Progress*, praises PHA for its various qualities which we will briefly discuss. Its major benefit is enhanced circulation, development of muscle endurance, and overall conditioning. It is known that the late Bruce Lee used a form of PHA to develop his exceptional muscularity and power (Whitley 1).

In his published and copyrighted paper "Peripheral Heart Action," Bob Gajda mentions that PHA will enhance the speed of blood circulation, facilitate muscle recovery by utilizing lower and upper leg exercises, and opposite function exercises (excerpt from Chapter III, "The Recovery Facilitation Factor").

UNILATERAL TRAINING

Another facet of the Krishna Warrior Fitness Challenge program is unilateral training, or moving a weight with one side of the body at a time (as opposed to bilateral training, or moving a weight with both sides of the body at a time). Unilateral form of training is an excellent way to overcome your plateaus and attain new levels of fitness. How so?

The unilateral way of exercising works not only the muscle itself but also on the nervous system. This is just as important as building the size of muscle cells. Training the nervous system allows one to trigger large and powerful muscle motor units. A motor unit is the primary structure in the development of force. To exert maximum force, you must turn on all of the motor units and keep them on for the longest time possible. In bilateral training, the nervous system does not turn on the motor units as much as in unilateral training. That means that you will not be as strong as you could become (Gamboa).

Each of us has a dominant body side, and when we move weights bilaterally, our stronger side will take over (especially with heavier weights). This may cause a disproportion in the size of muscle, strength, power, etc., thus, compromising your physical performance (Chernack 1). Exercising unilaterally will improve muscle symmetry. I personally worked with clients who corrected strength and mass differences between limbs.

San Diego State researchers found that unilateral form of training isolates muscles better by literally shocking them more, thus, resulting in quicker adaptation. It also increases blood flow as much as 50 to 100 percent more than in bilateral training. As some of you may already know, the greater the blood circulation, the more amino acids will be delivered to the working muscle, resulting in greater protein synthesis (Gamboa).

What is particularly interesting about unilateral training is that it helps bring the injured side back to a normal condition faster. Research shows that unilateral strength training produces increases in contralateral strength, or the inactive injured side (Munn 2). So if you have an injury in the right arm, you can still work your left arm and speed up right arm's recovery by improving its condition.

EXERCISES PRESENTED

Many of the exercises you are about to see and practice were independently developed and tested during my workouts, or workouts with my clients. Next to such exercises, I put a mark "ID," or "independently developed." That does not mean that the same or similar exercises don't exist elsewhere. Other exercises come from my practice of karate and may not be commonly known. Next to such exercises, I put a "K," for "karate." And still another group of exercises presented are progressions to already known exercises. These progressions were independently developed during my workouts or workouts with my clients. Next to such exercises, I put "IDP," or "Independently Developed Progression." *Very few times I include more than one progression for an exercise and thus the abbreviations will read as "IDP2" or "IDP3." Whenever the progression is not independently developed, I abbreviate it to a simple "P." When more such progressions are presented, I will number them as follows: P1, P2, etc.*

Many of the exercises presented I named after great warriors such as Arjuna, Bhishmadeva, etc., who appeared along with the Supreme Warrior Krishna on the battlefield of Kurukshetra 5,000 years ago. After all, they gave me their blessings and inspired me to compile this book, so I would like to humbly thank them. You can find brief biographies of those warriors in the Glossary section of this book. Pick your name from the list of warriors and use it for the duration of the training program (or beyond). Make sure you include the word *das* (servant) at the end of your chosen name to remain humble and allow the blessings of those great warriors to descend upon you.

MODIFIED EXERCISES

If you have certain limitations with range of motion or other kinds of health conditions, you should definitely consult your physician before attempting any of the exercises presented. The exercise modifications that are provided at the end of each exercise should be applied by those of you who experience either back, knee, or shoulder problems. You might be able to perform them safely because they ease stress on those areas, but they do not guarantee a complete risk-free exercise movement. Once again, consult your physician and/or use your own discretion. Only the exercises that put considerable stress on the lower back, knees, or shoulders were labeled "caution." Performing modified exercises will decrease the intensity of the exercise and the whole workout.

PERFORMANCE NUTRITION

As you may have heard, what you eat undoubtedly affects your physical performance. Not only that, but it even affects your mood. And you want to have the best mood possible for the workout, because it is not just a workout, it is The Workout of your life! That's right, the workout of your life, warriors. So we must try to maintain our machinery—body (with all its senses, brain, etc.)—in the best condition possible.

If your body is purified of toxic wastes, your body quickly learns how to perform at its optimal level. It will take some time to learn how to eat for optimum health and, if needed, for maximum performance. But, as with any science, the fitness of a Krishna warrior is a scientific process. Through gradual progression, you can attain to the highest performance level.

Set your own goals. I will give you a scheme, but you decide where you want to find yourself, say, a month or a year from today. This would be called a "training cycle." There will be goals for your body, for your mind, and for your spirit. The goals for your body will be divided into two: exercises and nutrition.

As most of us have lots of toxins to purge from our bodies, the first phase of nutrition is mostly cleansing. The second phase would deal more with optimizing your food intake for normal output work and then, peak output work—performing at your best. And unless you are a competitive athlete (or growing up or older) or are in the process of getting there, you might not need supplements other than a multivitamin and protein (whey, egg) designed for your needs.

Everybody, whether young or old, needs cleansing at the physical level, as well as the mental, intellectual, and spiritual level. Our bodies accumulate toxins, chemicals, and all sorts of bacteria from polluted air, food, and other people. All cleansing programs, such as the liver cleanse, juice fast, and water fast, have as their first requirement abstinence from flesh food (ESP 299–311). This cleanses not only the body but also the mind and intelligence. Eating light for optimum health (avoiding meat especially) and drinking purified water is the first step in rejuvenating your internal organs, such as the liver, kidneys, etc. This is what the Krishna Warrior Nutritional Program implements and puts emphasis on.

MEDITATIONAL TECHNOLOGIES

Delving into the depths of your inner self and emerging with a new, never before experienced sense of empowerment is the result of properly conducted meditation. When you begin your exercise with meditation, you take that mood or deep feeling into your workout to enhance performance.

I am sure that some of you might have practiced, seen, or at least read about many of them. In this book, I rely on three key meditational tools: sacred sound vibrations, sacred visual stimulation, and essential oils. Breathing and various postures and moves are of secondary importance, just because our workouts will serve as a dynamic form of meditation.

Sacred vibrations mean mantras, or powerful spiritual energies contained in sounds, that have a direct effect on your mind, emotions, and spirit. They come from ancient texts that describe powerful warriors who served the Supreme Warrior, or Krishna. You may feel free to use sacred sound vibrations from your own authorized scriptures.

Sacred visuals refer to pictures or paintings created based on descriptions found in ancient texts. They usually depict the Supreme Warrior Krishna in His different incarnations like Rama, Narasimha, Jesus Christ, Buddha, etc. Some of us may be very visual with photographic memories and may find ourselves more responsive to this kind of meditation.

Essential oils are therapeutic-grade substances obtained from plants, flowers, and trees. They are the essence, the life force of a plant, flower, or tree. Essential oils have been used for medicinal purposes since ancient times dating back to at least 4500 B.C. They are described in various scriptures such as the Bible, Vedas, etc.

Essential oils are different from common aromatic oils in that they are unadulterated, without any chemical additives or dilutions, and they meet high industry standards that qualify them as "therapeutic grade." Health professionals choose them to promote health. Essential oils have an effect on your threefold body: spirit, mind, and the physical body. They induce certain moods like courage, peace, love, clarity, focus, etc. We will avail ourselves of these oils before the meditation and the workout.

THE GORU PERSONALITY

Who is Goru? Goru is a fictitious person who I use as a literary device to make some important points in the mind and spirit sections of this book. He will ask typical questions and will get authorized answers from his teacher, that is, me. Goru is an aspiring warrior who decided to become a new person in body, mind, and spirit. You will have some fun listening to our conversations. And here is what he's got to say to you, potential Krishna warriors:

Hey, guys. This is me, Goru. I came out of nowhere, and Ark found me. I did not even know my name. He named me. Listen, by now I am almost done taking this intense Krishna warrior camp, and I feel like out of this world. I emerged with a rejuvenated body and mind. The feeling of empowerment, new ideas about my own life and its quality, feeling like I am in a new body, and, finally, the appreciation for my teacher's work now overflow my heart. All I can say is that once you follow the instructions of your Krishna warrior instructor, your life will never be the same; you will find yourself in a different world of transcendental fitness. You will know you are not this body but a spirit soul within. Yet because of this realization, you will actually do the best thing for your body, and you will try to do the best for others also. Friends, let's delve deep into the training mind-set and become the best we can be for ourselves, for our families, for the world, and for Krishna, the Supreme Warrior.

Arsenal One

Training

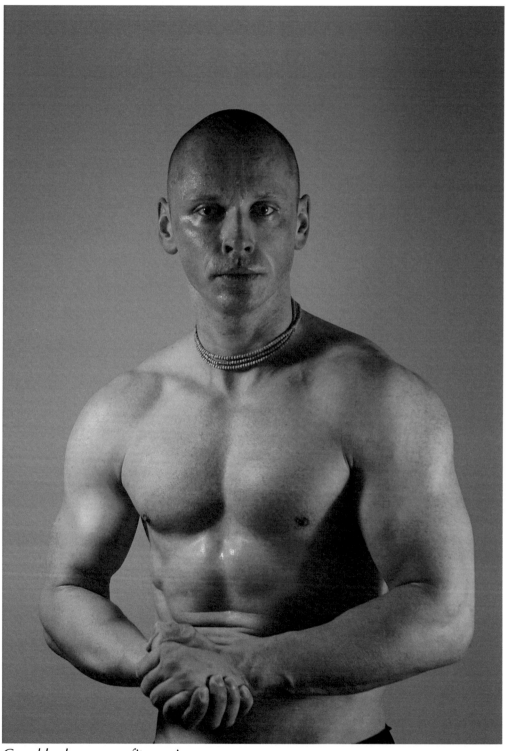

Good luck on your fitness journey

Chapter I

Beginner Krishna Warrior Program

He has been curiously watching me for a while. I was sitting almost motionlessly with closed eyes, chanting the holy mantras to myself. Finally, he said with a dose of impatience, "I can barely hear you . . . , Master."

I opened my eyes and concluded the meditation, putting my wooden beads in the chanting bag. "I am happy you are here . . . Thank you for visiting my humble institute." Standing up, I smiled and shook the boy's hand.

The boy pulled the chewing gum out of his mouth and put it in the wrapper for later use. His hands traveled to his pockets. His posture was not good, not healthy looking. After staring at me in a sort of disbelief, he said straightforwardly, "My folks sent me here to learn from you the way of life. They think I have problems that they can't solve, and they want me to be a successful man."

"So your parents care for you . . . Come on, sit down. Sit on the mat, here, next to the deity of Narasimha Deva," I motioned to him.

The boy looked at the great Narasimha Deva, the half-man, half-lion incarnation of Krishna, and hesitatingly sat down. "This . . ." he pointed to Narasimha Deva, "this you call Nara . . . Nara . . . sihhadev?"

"Yes, Narasimha Deva," I chuckled. "He came to Earth millions of years ago to rescue His devotee Prahlada. Pretty amazing, huh? Look at that mane, teeth, and claws, the emotion of supreme anger. See how powerful He looks." My heart started to beat faster when I described Narasimha Deva.

"Yeah, yeah . . . I see." He quickly looked at the other monuments and portraits that decorated the training hall of the institute. Then he looked at me. "So what are you going to teach me, Master?"

"First, do me a favor, would you? Don't call me 'Master.'" I looked at him somewhat intensely.

"Oh, really?" The boy scratched his head and looked at the wooden floor, thinking. "All right, Ark. So what do I have to do to . . . to be a better man, to be a warrior, to get over my challenges in school?"

"It's nice to have parents who care," I said.

"Ain't that right?"

"Good," I said quickly and stood up. "Do you want what your parents want for you?" I studied him.

"Well . . . no. I wish I could be stronger in body and, I guess, in mind. That is what we both agree on. But . . . I don't exactly want to be what they want me to be, like a lawyer of some sort, or a doctor. Dad is a lawyer, and he has his vision, but I have got mine too," the boy replied, nodding his head.

"What do you want to become?"

"I always wanted to be a firefighter," the boy's black eyes lit up.

"Great!" I exclaimed. "I will help you strengthen your body and mind, and then you will have the responsibility of using that power the way you would like, but in a positive, genuine way . . ." I paused.

"Got you, Ark," the boy looked up at me.

"We'll put you on a beginner's Character Evolution program. You'll develop patience, self-control, faith in your goal, determination, courage, and, finally, *power*. You like that?" I grabbed his hand with one hand and picked up a clipboard from the floor.

"Sounds interesting. There's some kind of energy . . . in this room. I sense it." He stood up very quickly and glanced at a portrait of Master *Prabhupada*. "I feel that what you're saying is going to happen."

"Yes. Your warrior name in this facility will be 'Goru.'" I jotted down his name and took his hand. "Let's go further into the training hall's chambers."

THE CASTLE OF MIND

"For him who has conquered the mind, the mind is the best of friends; but for one who has failed to do so, his mind will remain the greatest enemy."

Bhagavad-Gita 6.4

Goru was gasping for air, and his face expressed frustration. "Why don't I want to do this? Why am I struggling? I thought I would be a good student!"

"It's not you, Goru! Your mind, like a child, is protesting, because you perceive bodily pain. So the mind wants to reject it. But is the mind right?" I paused and bent down to be closer to Goru, who was attempting to execute another Crouching Tiger exercise.

"No, Ark, the stupid mind is *not* right. What should I go by when I am so tired that I only hear my mind?" His forehead was sweaty, and the whole floor around him was sprinkled with it.

"Normally, you should listen to your intelligence, but now it's hard to think logically and contact your intellect. Just keep your immediate goal in mind. Stay focused on the mission, boy!" I yelled back.

"Yeah! Focus on the mission. But I can't possibly do another hundred!" the boy barely got up and while kicking, lost his balance and fell to the floor on one knee. "Ouuch! Damn it!"

"No, that is yet another trick played by your mind! Disregard that baby mind. You are not a baby. Listen to the warrior within. Reach deep within yourself, Goru. Do your job as you planned. Come on, boy! Do you hear me? *Come on!*" I ran up close to Goru, got down, and yelled into his ear.

"Yeah! All right, I'll try." He got up awkwardly, his legs shivering from muscular fatigue. He was wobbling like a drunk.

"You must do it, boy. You're already determined, so half the battle is won. I know you will finish the workout." I checked my stopwatch. "You've got 80 left, Goru!"

SILVER DOOR 1: THE CASTLE OF INTELLIGENCE
REQUIRED ASSIGNMENTS

You are an aspiring Krishna warrior, and you are trying to ride the chariot of your body effectively and efficiently. The mind and intelligence are your reins and driver. You are the passenger. It is really up to you where and how you want to go. But you should educate your driver, because he is a beginner, just like you. You do not want to wreck the chariot of your body, do you? Here is the knowledge for you and the driver. Read on.

You must know what divine qualities make up a true warrior's character. Without exemplary character, there is no real power, no real health. The divine qualities are: steady determination, patience, self-control, fearlessness, courage, modesty, freedom from the passion for honor, freedom from anger, nonviolence, truthfulness, forgiveness, generosity, aversion to finding fault, gentleness, compassion for others, leadership.

As you may have noticed, some of these qualities are masculine and some are feminine. Whether you are a man or a woman, you must develop all of these. Your personality, your threefold body, will then be balanced. Real health means a balance of subtle and gross energies. Subtle matter and gross matter are interacting every minute and will affect your acts. They will affect your workout, too.

Have a notebook and devote a couple pages to each quality. You will set little daily and weekly goals to work on these traits of character (I'll leave it up to you how exactly you run your notebook). Little things build great things. Sure, you've heard that before.

Let's find something that would be an example of being self-controlled. For instance, not eating candy the whole day. If that is not difficult for you, then choose something else, like not watching TV for the whole day. The goals will vary, depending on your initial strengths and weaknesses. Then you move to the quality of generosity.

Let's say it is very hard for you to be generous with time given to people you don't spend a lot of time with, like your elderly neighbors. Often, you just barely notice them in the hallway, or when they slowly walk to the mailbox to pick up their mail. You may often just quickly say, "Hi, Mr. Morris," and don't care whether they answer or not. No wonder. These people are in a different age group. You just can't talk to them like you talk to your peers, your friends, colleagues at work. They may be boring, and you may feel like you have nothing in common. But quite often, they will become happy when they feel you really want to talk to them about something. They just require a different approach.

Resolve that when you see your elderly neighbor, you immediately wave your hand, smile, and loudly say, "Hi," or something like that. If they start talking to you, listen to them and take time out. Forget about what you have to do next just for a minute, or maybe for 2 or 3 minutes. Be generous with time you give to others. You will feel good afterward. Then you move on to patience.

Well, let's say that your elderly neighbor said, "Hi," first to you, and you replied the same, sending an automatic quick smile and barely making eye contact. You are hoping just to quickly move out of his or her way and go about your daily routine. STOP here. Stop your mind and your feet. And then when your neighbor notices that you stopped and made a long eye contact, he will start talking to you. Just listen and understand him. Have fun talking. Take time out of your daily routine. Be patient, even if something he or she is talking about seems so trivial to you.

So, warrior, you are supposed to be resourceful. I will let you go through all of these qualities and ponder each of them and how to develop them by being mindful of your daily thoughts, words, and actions. Find an example of how each quality would practically be demonstrated by you in real life and how it would not be.

For me, courage may not mean the same as for you. I am afraid of things that you probably would laugh off. Thus, our daily, weekly assignments will differ. Find something challenging to work on every day. Every time you succeed in a situation, you write a "plus" or "check" in your Krishna warrior notebook. Date it. Track everything. If for 1 week you did everything well on a particular quality, give yourself a star.

BRONZE DOOR 1
ASSIGNMENTS:

1. (Required) Go to Chapter 4 (Nutrition) and find your body type.
2. (Required) Adjust your food intake accordingly. Make a shopping list that reflects your body type.
3. (Required) Perform a fitness assessment on yourself, or have someone do it for you to find out your starting weight, your body fat percentage, and your lean body weight (muscle, bones, water). Write everything down in your diary or on your Personal Achievement Goal Sheet (see Chapter 5/Physical Assessments).
4. (Required) Start going through a preliminary cleansing phase.[1] To do that, follow your body type diet and abstain from all flesh food. If you are not prepared to do that, then consume flesh food only once a day at around noon (when your digestive acid is very strong). Consume more vegetables and fruits. Use lemon essential oil[2] with any water you drink.
5. (Required) Fill out your Personal Achievement Goal Sheet for the first month and obtain color note cards (see Chapter 5). Have one of your family members or training

buddies check on you before every workout and collect a card from you. You should turn in a card every time you do the KWFC workout (three times a week). At the end of the workout, your friend should give you a reward (it could be a bottle of organic juice, a coupon to Whole Foods store, or anything positive and conducive to further training) or a punishment (e.g., 1,000 push-ups a day).

6. (Optional) Write out your daily schedule with, most importantly, workout times and workout types included. If you want, you can get as specific as you want with your daily schedule and follow some of the schedules that I provided for different body types.

7. (Optional) Create and start filling out your Personal Record Sheet (see Chapter 5).

GOLDEN DOOR: MEDITATION[3]

1. Put aside distracting thoughts for a moment and kneel, heels under your buttocks. When you cross your feet, the right foot should rest on top of the left. Your palms may rest on your thighs. Or, assume the following hand position: put your loosely clenched left fist in your right palm. The thumbs of both hands should point upward and be joined. If you choose this hand position, rest your hands on your upper thighs. The third variation is to interlock your fingers and assume the same upward thumb position. Finally, straighten your spine and half-close your eyes.

2. Next, visualize your favorite authorized form of the Supreme Warrior, Krishna (God), and become consciously surrendered to Him in all your bodily and mental functions. You may at this time close your eyes completely. You can also quietly chant the name of the Supreme Warrior, God, in the language of your own scriptures (Allah, Jesus Christ, Krishna, Buddha, etc.).

3. While keeping your eyes closed (or half-closed), stretch your arms out in front of you and, as you bring the palms of your extended hands back to your chest, inhale to the limit of your lung capacity. By the time your hands travel to the sides of your chest, flex them to form fists (palms facing up). While inhaling, become aware that you are absorbing the dazzling yellow light[4] emanating from the Supreme Warrior. Accept it as a gift.

Hold your breath for a few seconds and, while shooting out your hands horizontally, rapidly release the air and open your hands. Your attention should now be absorbed in returning all your energy to its source, the Supreme Warrior.

After the primary release, while you still have some air left to exhale, slowly draw a circle with your palms facing out (arms held in air in an outstretched position). This slow motion will emphasize the pacifying desire to return all energy to the Supreme Warrior. Thus, with every inhalation, you are blissfully accepting the Lord's energy to enter your body, and upon exhalation, returning that energy to him without attachment and with pleasure. Continue with such transcendental breathing for 1 or 2 minutes.

4. Return to the hand position from step 1.

Fully surrendered and detached from the results of your actions, jump to your feet from the kneeling position, or rhythmically stand up, and perform your martial duty as well as you can for Lord Krishna's pleasure. Be one in spirit with Arjuna and the other Lord's eternal warriors!

At the end of the session, repeat the sequence, but change step 3 (see ending meditation) and 5.

WORKOUT PLAN

Warm-up. Duration of about 5 minutes. Apply Peppermint essential oil[5] to your temples, forehead, and cheeks and then inhale it at least 10 times for increased stimulation of the mind. Make sure you do not apply it too closely to the eyes as it will burn.

Equipment needed: Stepper

Presenter: Warrior Kim D.

Execution:
Position the stepper to your side. Do a side step from one side of the stepper to another (See Photos X.1–3), then immediately hit the floor (get in a push-up position) and perform one somewhat fast push-up, followed by a Mountain Climber (switch legs three times). See Photos X.4–5. Then immediately stand up and do another side step. Then another push-up and a Mountain Climber of three and so on. While doing this, you have the option of turning toward the stepper (after crossing it) and doing push-ups on its edge (as shown in the pictures) or having the stepper always to your side and doing push-ups on the floor.

Comments: Start with a medium tempo and after a couple of minutes, begin moving faster. Push-ups can be fast in the beginning. Mountain Climbers should be performed at a medium tempo in the beginning. Watch your feet initially until you get the hang of the side step. DO NOT cross your feet.

Progression:
Hold a 5-pound dumbbell in each hand while doing this warm-up. When you do push-ups, you use dumbbells as your support instead of the stepper.

Perform a military press with two dumbbells immediately after standing up from the Mountain Climber. Quickly tap two or three times on the floor with the foot that ends up being further away from the stepper after completing your side step.

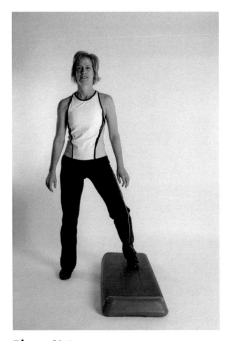

Photo X.1

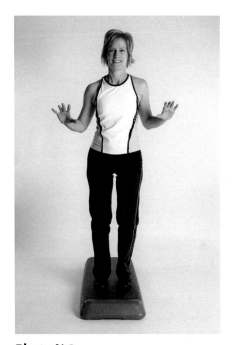

Photo X.2

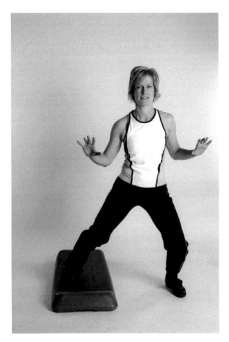

Photo X.3

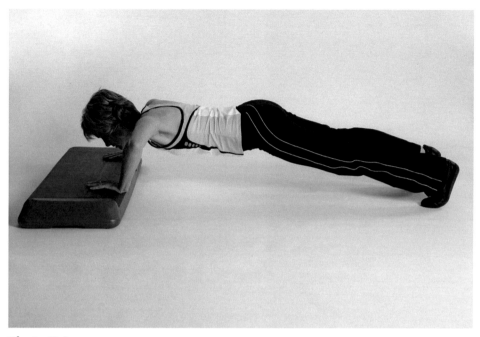

Photo X.4

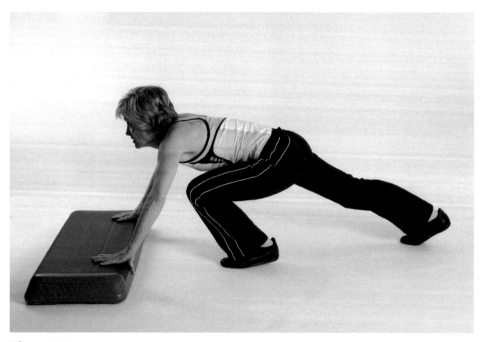

Photo X.5

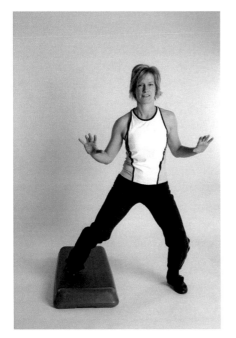

Photo X.6

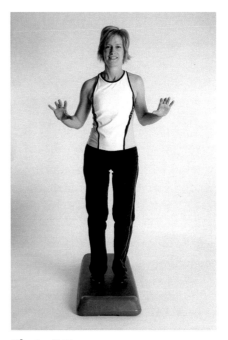

Photo X.7

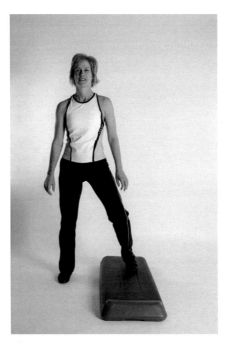

Photo X.8

EXERCISES IN THE MAIN CORE OF THE WORKOUT

Equipment needed:
A mat, adjustable cable station, a stepper with at least one riser, light or medium elastic band, two pair of light to medium dumbbells or plates, a rope (as used on cable stations for Triceps Pressdowns), a towel, a stopwatch.

Estimated Completion Time (ECT): 40 minutes

General Comments:
ECT listed above was calculated during a rather medium-paced workout with short breaks (30 seconds) after each sequence to catch your breath and adjust equipment for the upcoming sequence. Meditation, warm-up, and cooldown times are not included. If you go over 40 minutes, then you probably rested too long between exercises and/or sequences. Remember, the idea behind the PHA system of training is to go NONSTOP. For a competitive completion time of the beginner's workout with my own loading parameters, see Chapter 5, Physical Assessments.

SEQUENCE 1 (REPEATED THREE TIMES IN A CIRCUITLIKE FASHION):
Alternating Push-ups

Reverse Swimmers

Sahadeva's Rocking Chair

One-legged Hip-ups

Monster Jump

SEQUENCE 2 (REPEATED THREE TIMES IN A CIRCUITLIKE FASHION):
Push-up Walk-over Stepper

Yudhisthira's Row

Fighting Yaksha

Rakshasa Squats

SEQUENCE 3 (REPEATED THREE TIMES IN A CIRCUITLIKE FASHION):
Arjuna's Bow

Hanuman's Extension

Bhishmadeva's Running Wild Row

Karate Squats

DESCRIPTIONS OF EXERCISES IN THE BEGINNER'S PROGRAM, SEQUENCE 1
Alternating Push-ups

Difficulty level: I

Origin: IDP

Presenter: Warrior Bill

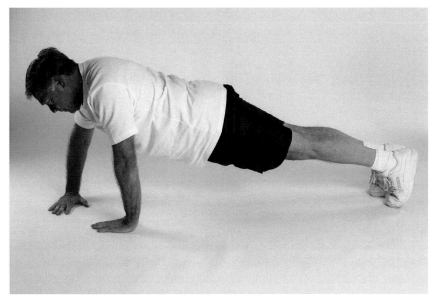

Photo 1.1

Starting position:
It is said that push-ups are the best exercises for the upper body. And it is quite true. While pushing off with your arms and working them, you also contract the whole torso (abdominal muscles, back extensors, oblique muscles, and even legs). In this particular push-up, you position your right arm in front in such a way that the palm is roughly on the level of your head and turned in (see Photo 1.1).

Movement:
As you push off the floor, the right arm will bend out so that elbow will go out to form a 90-degree angle between the forearm and biceps (see Photo 1.2). The other arm is down

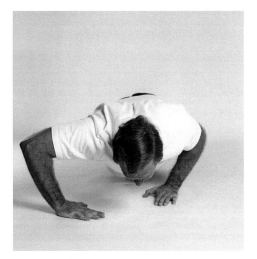

Photo 1.2

low next to your side. As you push off the floor, this arm will brush against your side. As you do alternating push-ups, you can switch hand positions on every repetition, or you can first do seven or eight push-ups on your left side and then switch and do an equal number of push-ups in the alternate position.

Major muscles involved:
The work of the left arm focuses on the triceps brachii (back of arm) muscle, which assists the pectoralis muscle (chest) in the exercise. The other arm will work in just the same way as in

a regular push-up and will, thus, work the pectoralis muscles (the prime mover muscle), the anterior deltoid (front shoulder, assisting mover), and the triceps brachii (assisting mover).

Ark's tips:
Keep your abdominals tight and slightly pushed in. Ensure that you are not hyperextending your back. Each time you push off the floor, try to consciously contract the muscles in your hand (fingers included) just as if you wanted to tear out a piece of the floor. This will ensure that more neural signals will be sent from the smaller muscles in your hand to the larger muscles in your arm and torso.

Breathing technique:
Exhale when pushing up and inhale on your way back.

Sports applications:
This type of push-up strengthens the arms in positions that are very specific to hand positions of some blocks found in certain martial arts such as karate. It is a good triceps isolating exercise; therefore, it is especially beneficial for martial artists of various kinds and/or athletes whose disciplines involve pushing motions.

Come on, warrior, you're not done yet!/progression:

IDP2:
As you lower your upper body, lift up the foot (keep the leg straight) on the side of the hand that's close to your body. Wait until you complete the pushing-up motion, then switch feet.

> Reverse Swimmers
> Difficulty level: I
> Origin: IDP
> Presenter: Self

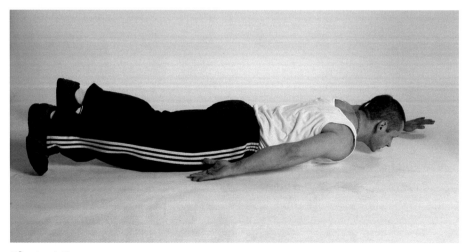

Photo 1.3

Starting position:

Lie on your stomach on the mat with your right arm alongside your body and the other extended in front (see Photo 1.3).

Movement:

Contract your abdominal and lower back muscles simultaneously, lifting your chest and both arms off the mat. Start moving your extended arm out to the side in a circular swimminglike motion (see Photos 1.4–7). At the same time, you should be turning your head in the direction of your circling arm and looking over that shoulder. Bring the arm to your side and back in front of you. Rest your chest and knees on the mat for a split second. Repeat. Perform 15 of these Swimmers and switch sides.

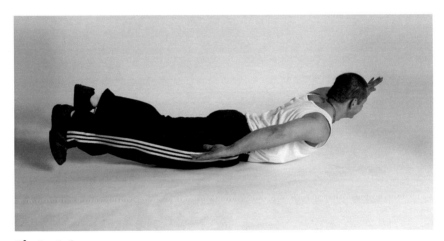

Photo 1.4

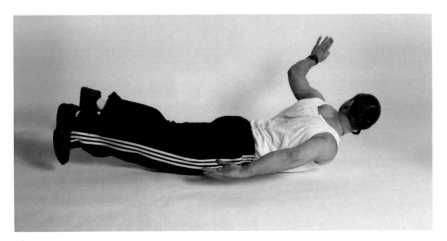

Photo 1.5

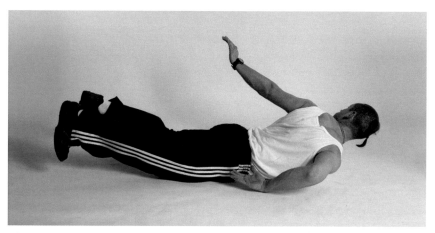

Photo 1.6

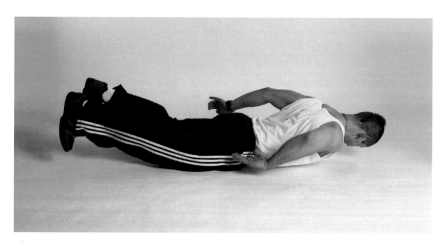

Photo 1.7

Major muscles involved:
The muscles acting here are erector spinae (lower back), latissimus dorsi (performs the twist-ing motion), the internal and external obliques (perform the twisting motion), upper and lower trapezius, posterior deltoid (rear shoulder which is the prime mover for the arm), and rectus abdominis (stabilizes your body to allow twisting). To engage your gluteus maximus and biceps femoris (hamstring), keep your knees off the mat for the duration of the set.

Ark's tips:
Divide the whole movement into four phases: lifting up, twisting, untwisting, then going down. Make sure to perform this exercise slowly, pausing for a second after every phase of the movement except for the "staying down" phase. This will ensure that your back muscles (and others) stay under optimal tension.

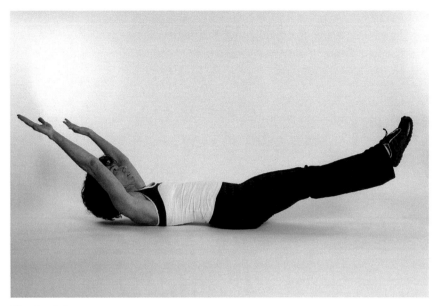

Photo 1.8

Breathing technique:
As you are lifting your chest off the floor, exhale halfway, hold your breath, and pause for a second. Then turn, look over your left shoulder (if you are working on your left side), and exhale the rest of the air.

Sports applications:
This is good for any kind of sport that requires torso twisting. Swimmers especially can benefit from this exercise. It's a great exercise for improving posture.

Come on, warrior, you're not done yet!/progression:

IDP2:
Break down the exercise into phases of moving and holding. After lifting the upper body, hold the position for 5 seconds, then twist and hold your position for 5 more seconds. Next, untwist and hold the upper body in an up position for 5 seconds, and then start twisting again. So here you never touch your chest to the floor during the set but maintain constant levels of concentric and isometric tension.

Sahadeva's Rocking Chair

Difficulty level: I

Caution: If you have back problems, you may be able to perform the exercise modification provided.

Origin: K

Presenter: Warrior Susan

Starting position:

Lie down on a mat with arms extended above the head and legs straight. Lift your legs and arms off the mat (see Photo 1.8). You will notice that your whole abdominal area tightens up. Your butt should also tighten up.

Movement:

Using kinetic momentum, start rocking on your butt so that when your shoulder blades touch the mat, your legs are up in the air, and when your feet touch the floor, your

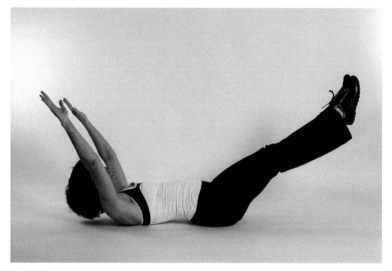

Photo 1.9

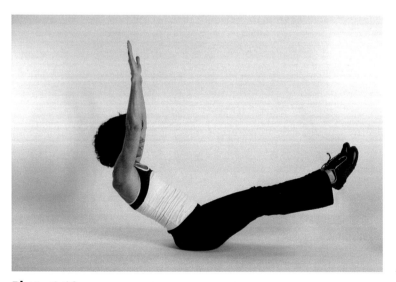

Photo 1.10

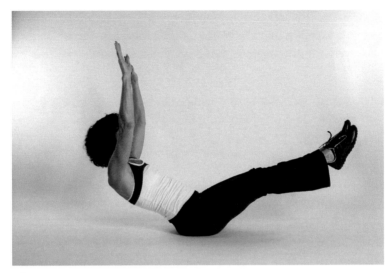

Photo 1.11

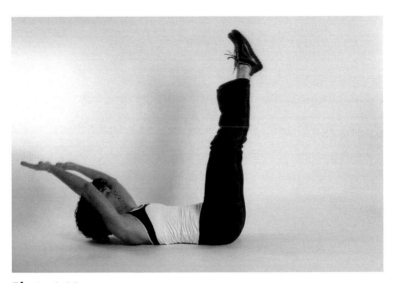

Photo 1.12

shoulder blades and back are up in the air (see Photos 1.9–12). Continue in this manner for 15 repetitions.

Major muscles involved:
The muscles are contracting isometrically, which means that they are neither shortening nor lengthening. Nevertheless, heat is being produced and work is performed. You will feel it! The majority of work is performed here by rectus abdominis, the main core stabilizing muscle, transversus abdominis, the gluteus, and the oblique muscles.

Ark's tips:
When executing this exercise, make sure not to bend your legs too much as this will compromise the effectiveness of the exercise. Keep your arms above and behind your head.

Breathing technique:
Inhale air while rocking back and exhale while rocking forward. Alternatively, you could exhale while rocking back and inhale rocking forward.

Sports applications:
This exercise can help athletes in different sports such as volleyball when performing a spike. Other disciplines such as basketball can also benefit from the Rocking Chair as they require jumping in the air, twisting the torso at the same time, and shooting the ball or fighting for it. The core is often partially contracted in such air battles, and the transverse abdominis muscle is used in sports with short-term power activities; it pulls abs inward, forcing exhalation. Practitioners of football and martial arts such as karate will greatly benefit from the exercise.

Come on, warrior, you're not done yet!/progression:

IDP1:
Place a 5-pound dumbbell between your feet (hold it tight while rocking). To counterbalance your body, also hold a 5-pound plate in both hands.

Modification (extension-biased persons[6]):
Bend legs at the knees and arms at the elbows. This will round your back a little. You could also hold onto your knees with your hands for more support and the lessening of the back extension involved here.

> One-legged Hip-ups
>
> Difficulty level: B
>
> Origin: ID
>
> Presenter: Warrior Kim D.

Starting position:
Place yourself on a mat on the back with legs bent at the knees. Then lift up one leg off the mat and keep it straight (but not locked). See Photo 1.13.

Movement:
Press firmly into the ground with your other foot and lift the small of your back off the mat (push your hips up). You will feel tension in the hamstring muscles (back of leg) and both biceps femoris and semitendinosus. Keep lifting both hips up until your upper thigh of the supporting leg and your torso form a straight line (see Photo 1.14). The other leg is up in the air, aligned at the thigh with the supporting leg. Hold the tension for half a second or slightly longer and bring your hips down on the mat again. Repeat 15 times for each leg. You can also push off from the heel of the supporting leg to put more emphasis on the hamstring group of muscles.

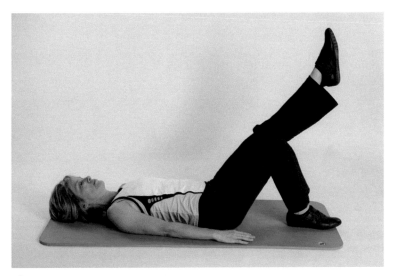

Photo 1.13

Major muscles involved:
In addition to your hamstring muscles, gluteus maximus is at work here, as well as erector spinae.

Ark's tips:
The key to performing Hip-ups with greatest effectiveness is accelerating the movement at first and, once in the up position, holding the position for a second and contracting your muscles as hard as you can.

Breathing technique:
Exhale on your way up and breathe in on your way down.

Sports applications:
Hip-ups are great for strengthening your lower back muscles, upper legs, and butt. Often in sports such as basketball and volleyball, an athlete will assume a hyperextended position in the air, as in spiking, for example. In a spike, the abdominal muscles would extend, the spine would hyperextend, and the back muscles would contract. An instant later, the muscles will pull in the opposite direction to hit the volleyball. The Hip-ups will strengthen these muscles in a sport-specific way.

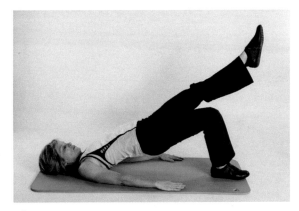

Photo 1.14

Come on, warrior, you're not done yet!/progression:

IDP1:
Place a 10-pound weight on your hip bone of the leg that's pushing off the floor.

> Monster Jump/Single-legged Explosion
>
> Difficulty level: B
>
> Origin: ID
>
> Presenter: Warrior Kim D.

Starting position:
Stand on a flat concrete surface with your right leg forward and bent. Left leg is straight and either flat or heel is off the floor to prepare for exploding. Hands can be kept bent in front of you or alongside your body. See Photo 1.15.

Movement:
Commence the exercise by rapidly pushing off of your right leg and jumping up as high as you can (see Photos 1.16–18). Land on the right foot first, then the toes of left foot will touch the floor. Reload and explode up again.

Major muscles involved:
In this Monster Jump, you work fast and twitch fibers in the legs. Muscles such as the front and back of the thighs (quadriceps and hamstring group) do the majority of the work. The soleus muscles in the calf are assisting the larger muscles in the upper leg to execute the jump. Lower back (erector spinae) and abdominal muscles (rectus abdominis) work as well to aid primarily in stabilization and balancing the body during takeoff and landing.

Ark's tips:
Make sure that you land first on the ball of the right foot and then your shift weight to the rest of the foot and the left leg. This ensures the cushioning necessary to protect your joints and ligaments in such an explosive exercise. As you jump up, look up and ahead to see the environment to retain a good sense of orientation and dynamic balance. Then as you come down, you should lower your chin a little to be able to see the environment at a lower level to help in landing your leg.

Breathing technique:
Exhale as you push off and inhale as you come down.

Sports applications:
Runners, and especially sprinters (who push off), will benefit from the Monster Jump because it improves hip joint flexibility. Other sports that will find the exercise beneficial are racquetball, fencing, basketball, football (tackling), gymnastics (when doing Chinese Splits), and ballet. Some kicks in the martial arts, such as taekwondo or karate, may require jumping up high from a normal or low position and landing in a balanced fighting stance.

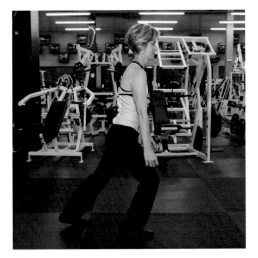

Photo 1.15

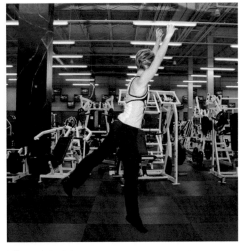

Photo 1.16

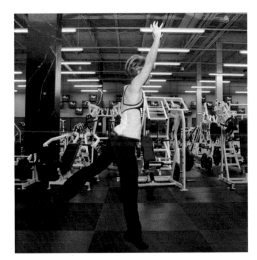

Photo 1.17

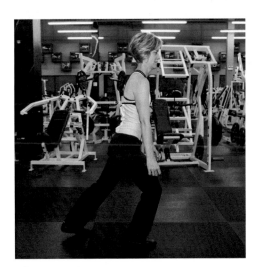

Photo 1.18

As such, the Monster Jump will be beneficial, especially for taekwondokas, who are known for their jumping-in-the-air kicks.

Come on, warrior, you're not done yet!/progression:

IDP1:
Grab a 10-pound plate and hold it close to your chest. It is very good to cross your arms around the plate to ensure it doesn't move along with your arms and, thus, create unnecessary stress on the lower back.

Okay, now let's repeat this sequence twice more before we start sequence 2.

DESCRIPTIONS OF EXERCISES IN THE BEGINNER'S PROGRAM, SEQUENCE 2

Push-up Walk-over Stepper

Difficulty level: I

Origin: IDP

Presenter: Warrior Greg

Starting position:

Place a stepper with the long side toward your side. Position yourself in a push-up position with the stepper next to your side (see Photo 1.19).

Movement:

Perform a regular push-up and then walk over the stepper (see Photos 1.20–22) to the other side and do another push-up. Then walk over to the other side and do another push-up. Perform at least 20 push-ups in this manner. As you walk over the stepper, starting with your right side, be cautious to first place your right hand somewhere in the middle of the stepper and then the right foot. Next, bring your left hand and foot so that your whole body is in on the stepper in a push-up position. But do not do the push-up yet. Go to the other side of the stepper by repeating the same movement. Once you are on the other side, do your push-up and then come back on the stepper and to its left side starting with your right side.

Major muscles involved:

The Walk-over exercise works muscles such as the pectoralis (chest) and triceps brachii. But in addition to that, it strengthens your abdominals as well as wrists and muscles of your hand because of the way you reposition your body on the stepper.

Ark's tips:

Tighten up your wrists and hands when walking over the stepper. This contraction of your hands and wrists will reinforce further muscular adaptation in the muscles connecting your hand and forearm.

Breathing technique:

Exhale when walking over the stepper. Once you are on the other side of the stepper, inhale and go down into a push-up position. Perform a fast push-up while breathing out. Inhale quickly, and as soon as your hands are touching the stepper, again start exhaling.

Sports applications:

This exercise is great for sports requiring strong wrists and core, especially disciplines involving all sorts of pushing, holding (boxing, football, judo), and balancing on the bar (gymnastics). It specifically improves strength endurance of the arm in the extended range of motion (when you are constantly moving over the stepper and holding your body in a push-up position).

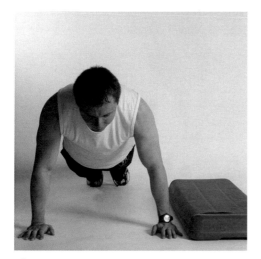

Photo 1.19

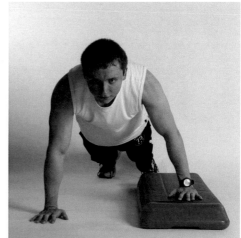

Photo 1.20

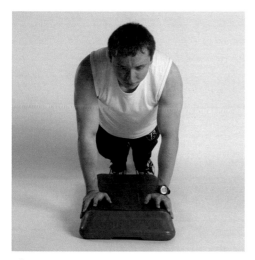

Photo 1.21

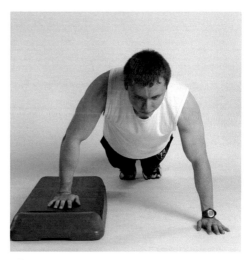

Photo 1.22

Come on, warrior, you're not done yet!/progression:

IDP2:

Lift up one foot as you go down and hold it in the air until the Push-up is completed. Lift up the foot that's further from the stepper.

Yudhisthira's Row/Squat, Reverse Sit-up, and Row

Difficulty level: I

Origin: ID

Presenter: Warrior Kim G.

Starting position:

This is another total body exercise that offers the benefit of squats, sit-ups, and seated rows. For this, you will need a cable station that adjusts. Adjust the pulley so that it is well above your head. Hold on to a bar that you ordinarily use for rows (your cable station should allow you to switch between different pieces, such as triangle bar, straight bar, square handle, etc.) with your hands extended straight in front of you and down (see Photo 1.23). Adjust the weight on the pulley so that you will be able to perform a Squat and a sit-down on a mat without the weight pulling you up (obviously the weight should be less than your total body weight).

Movement:

While holding the bar carefully, squat down and go even lower to sit down on a mat (see Photos 1.24–25). Tighten up your core and then lean back to touch the mat with your back (Reverse Sit-up). Come back to almost a straight sitting position and perform a rowing motion (see Photo 1.26). Make sure you do not lean too far, though; your elbows should not touch the floor at the end of the rowing motion. Next, extend your arms back out in front of you, lean forward with your torso, and while generating kinetic momentum, stand up on your feet (see Photos 1.27–28) back to your starting position. Once again, the weight on the pulley should be adjusted in such a way that it will help you get up, but it will provide a significant resistance for your rowing motion to occur. You should be able to perform 15 repetitions of this complex movement, and it should get your heart rate up quite a bit!

Major muscles involved:

Muscles used in this movement are leg and core muscles, such as rectus femoris, vastus medialis, rectus abdominis, as well as arms and back, biceps brachii, and latissimus dorsi.

Ark's tips:

This exercise is dynamic in nature. Therefore, you will need to squat down fast, pull on the bar and get down on the mat fast. At the same time, do not go too fast so that your good form is sacrificed. Learn the exercise first at a slow or medium tempo, and then gradually increase speed.

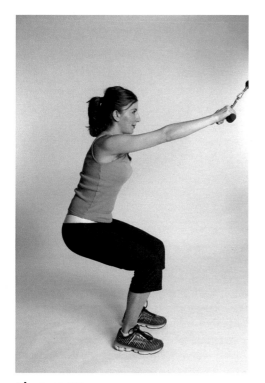

Photo 1.23

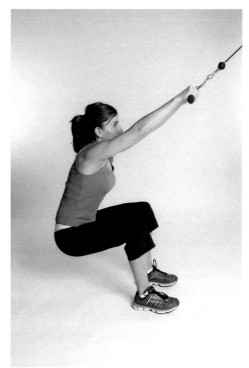

Photo 1.24

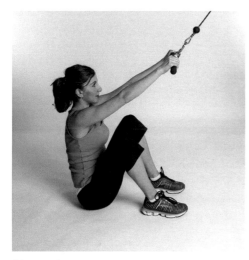

Photo 1.25

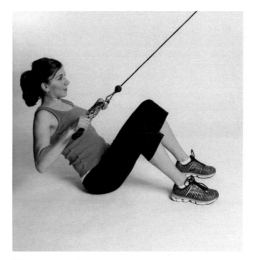

Photo 1.26

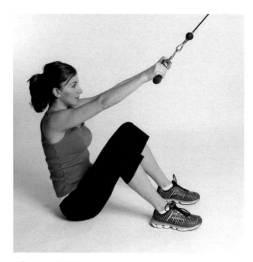

Photo 1.27

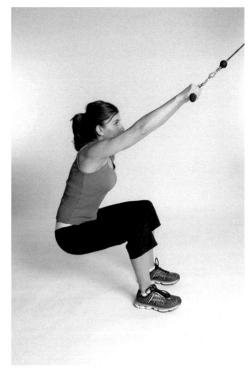

Photo 1.28

Breathing technique:
Begin exhaling when squatting down. The final portion of your exhalation should happen at the time of rowing. Next, while extending your arms to a straight position and coming forward with your torso, rapidly inhale. By the time your feet are flat on the floor and before you squat back up, rapidly exhale. Take a fast breath and start exhaling and squatting again.

Sports applications:
The Squat, Reverse Sit-up, and Row complex of exercises is great for a total body anaerobic endurance workout. You could have a great 10-minute workout doing this one exercise, and it is sure to activate most muscles in your body. Working legs, torso, and arms, the exercise will pump the blood up and down your whole body, increasing the cardio effect of the workout. It's great for sports that involve rowing, such as canoeing, kayaking, etc.

Come on, warrior, you're not done yet!/progression:

IDP1:
After you do the Reverse Sit-up, raise both of your legs and do the Row. Try to keep your legs straight.

Fighting Yaksha/Bicycle with Bands

Difficulty level: I

Caution: If you have back problems, you may be able to perform the exercise modification provided.

Origin: ID

Presenter: Warrior Rich

Starting position:
Attach a light or medium tension tube to a pulley station. Lie down on a mat with feet toward the pulley station. Hold the two handles of the rubber tube with each hand (palms-down grip). Lift your left leg up and straighten it out. Lift your right leg off the floor, but bend it at the knee (heel of your foot should stay a couple inches off the floor). See Photo 1.29. Raise your right arm holding the band over your head so that it is approximately 8–12 inches from the floor (the palm of right hand will be up). See Photo 1.30. Make sure that there is enough tension in the right side of the tube (for a front raise which will work your shoulder muscle). If there isn't, then move the mat further away from the pulley station.

Movement:
Bend your left leg, simultaneously straightening out the right one as you bring your right arm down and left up (see Photo 1.31). The whole motion occurs simultaneously. Perform 15 Fighting Yakshas.

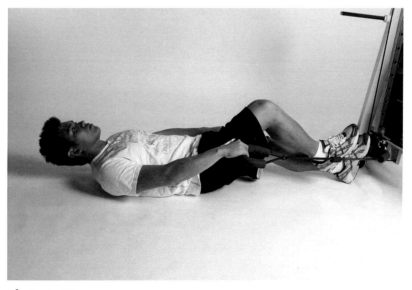

Photo 1.29

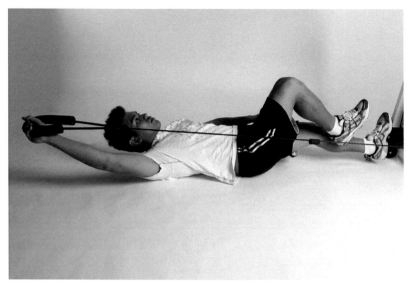

Photo 1.30

Major muscles involved:
In the upper body, you have the anterior deltoid (front shoulder) at work. In the core and lower body, you have rectus abdominis (abdominals), pectineus, tensor fasciae latae (hip flexors), and upper rectus femoris (front of thigh) working.

Ark's tips:
Focus on maintaining muscle tension in the abdominal area. You should really start feeling the pull in the front shoulder from almost the beginning of the arm raise. If you don't, you should, as mentioned before, move yourself further away from the pulley station. Don't use a thick band, as you will not be able to do the movement correctly.

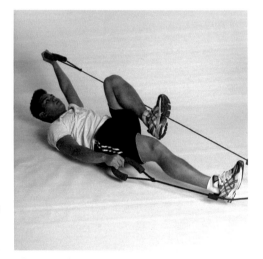

Photo 1.31

Breathing technique:
Exhale as you bring your left arm and leg up. Then inhale quickly and start exhaling as you bring the right arm and leg up.

Sports applications:
The Fighting Yaksha will prove effective for those who play sports that require moving arms up and in front, such as basketball, volleyball (e.g., blocking), diving, boxing, and

karate (e.g., in the uppercut). As far as the lower body is concerned, gymnasts, martial artists, runners, and soccer players, among others, should perform the Fighting Fly because of the need for abdominal strength to lift up the legs to a 90-degree angle or more. For example, runners could increase their stride length and kickers could lift legs and thighs more forward to deliver powerful kicks.

Come on, warrior, you're not done yet!/progression:

IDP1:
Use angle weights to increase tension on the legs and hips for the bicycle part of the Fighting Yaksha.

Modification (extension-biased persons[7]):
Place your arms on the mat alongside your body and press down firmly for more back support. Perform the Leg Bicycle. When you are done, immediately bend both legs at the knees and press your heels down into the floor. Grab both elastic bands and perform alternated raises as described above.

Rakshasa Squat/Fast Squats with Arms Punching Up

Difficulty level: B

Origin: IDP

Presenter: Warrior Bill

Starting position:
Stand in a partial squat position with your feet placed shoulder width apart and toes pointed straight ahead. Keep your arms out in front of you, bent at approximately a 90-degree angle (see Photo 1.32).

Movement:
Commence the movement by rapidly straightening the legs out. As you quickly come out of the squat position, push both of your hands forcefully up until they completely straighten out (see Photo 1.33). Quickly squat down until your thighs are almost parallel with the floor (push your hips back as if sitting on an imaginary chair that was placed behind you), thus, returning to a starting position. You will notice how your back will slightly arch and tighten up.

Major muscles involved:
As you flex your knee, the rectus femoris (front of thigh) does the majority of the work. Assisting in the movement are: biceps femoris (back of thigh) and gluteus maximus (butt). The erector spinae (lower back), rectus abdominis (stomach), as well as external obliques (sides) contract isometrically to stabilize the torso. When you punch, the upper body anterior deltoid, pectoralis muscles, as well as triceps brachii are the prime and assisting movers. In the quick returning of the arms, latissimus dorsi plays the most important role.

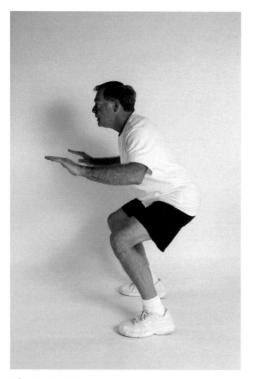

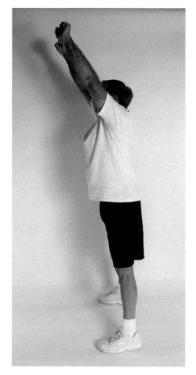

Photo 1.32   **Photo 1.33**

Ark's tips:
To do this exercise correctly, you already need to be familiar with correct squatting. If you are not, then start out with slow squats in front of the mirror so you can master the proper form. Shift your weight to the heels as you squat down. Focus on exploding your hands up as fast as you can just as if you were punching. It helps if you flex your fists at the end of the punch. As you return, open them up slightly and explode up. Flex them again in the up position.

Breathing technique:
Inhale as you squat and exhale as you come out of the squat position. The final exhalation should take place when you punch up.

Sports applications:
Squats will help in performing basic sport skills, such as high or distance jumping, kicking techniques, running, skipping, and lifting or pushing with the legs. Anybody who plays basketball, volleyball, soccer, football, runs, or practices martial arts will benefit from this squat. In addition, the punching-up action will, when done correctly, improve the speed of your punches.

Come on, warrior, you're not done yet!/progression:

IDP2:

Stand between a low cable pulley station so that you have a handle on both sides of you. Grab the two handles and perform a Rakshasa Squat with added weight.

Okay, now, let's repeat this sequence twice more before we start sequence 3.

DESCRIPTIONS OF EXERCISES IN THE BEGINNER'S PROGRAM, SEQUENCE 3

Arjuna's Bow/Stringing the Bow

Difficulty level: B

Origin: ID

Presenter: Warrior Bill

Starting position:

Stand with your feet approximately shoulder width apart, slightly turned out. Hold tightly a medium- to high-tension elastic band in front of you (see Photo 1.34).

Movement:

Raise your arms to about shoulder height. Stretch the band by extending your left arm out in front of you while pulling the other arm back (see Photos 1.35–37). The movement should resemble stringing a bow. String 15 times on each side.

Major muscles involved:

This exercise is great for shoulders, particularly the posterior deltoid (rear shoulder) of the arm that's moving back and the anterior deltoid (front shoulder) of the arm moving forward. In addition, you improve the strength of muscles in the palm, wrist (pronator quadratus), and forearm (e.g., extensor carpi). The work of these muscles in the stringing motion is predominantly isometric (the muscle is not shortening or lengthening). Back muscles such as the trapezius are involved in the concentric contraction (the rearing up motion). The biceps brachii is involved in both arms as an assisting muscle (in the rearing up arm) and a stabilizing muscle (in the arm stretching forward).

Ark's tips:

Initiate a steady, controlled movement. Believe that you are actually on the battlefield stringing that bow! Try to flex all the muscles in the arms. Keep the wrists of both hands locked/straight. Turn your hand toward the hand that's moving forward and look at your fist. Once you've strung the bow and your arms are straight, you can hold that position for at least a second. Return the same way. You can do this exercise in two ways. One is that you hold your front arm extended throughout the set and only your rear arm is stringing the band. The second way is that both arms are extending the band; one arm travels forward and the other travels back.

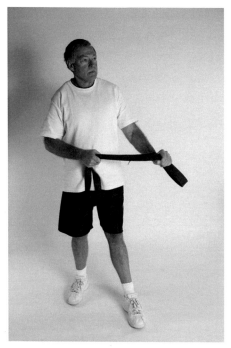

Photo 1.34

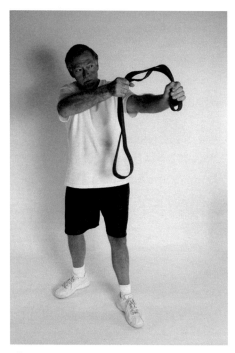

Photo 1.35

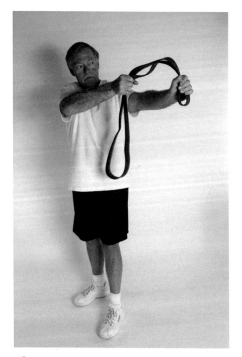

Photo 1.36

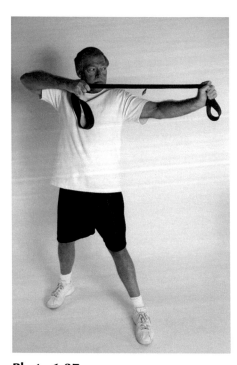

Photo 1.37

Breathing technique:
Exhale when stretching the band and inhale when pulling it back.

Sports applications:
Archery! You are more than welcome to follow in the footsteps of a great Krishna warrior, Arjuna, the superarcher. This exercise will help you in that discipline. The muscles involved here will help any athlete or person who practices punching and pushing sports, such as kickboxing, boxing, wrestling, etc.

Come on, warrior, you're not done yet!/progression:

P1:
As you stretch the bend with your right hand, also step back and to the right with your right leg. The leg should end up in a locked position, and the foot should be turned out at approximately 45 degrees in relation to left foot (see demo video). After completing the stringing movement, return your right foot close to your left foot (closer than shown in the starting position).

IDP1:
You can raise the back leg and perform the same exercise.

> Hanuman's Extension/Suspended Triceps Extension
>
> Difficulty level: A
>
> Origin: IDP
>
> Presenter: Warrior Greg

Starting position:
Find a stable end of a bar and hook a rope or your towel around it. Firmly grab the two ends of the rope and move your feet back and place them shoulder width apart (see Photo 1.38). Contract muscles in the hands, arms, abdominals, and legs.

Movement:
Shifting most of the weight to your arms, literally rest on the rope and begin bending them at the elbows until your head goes under the bar and your biceps and forearm touch (see Photos 1.39–40). As you do so, try to keep the elbows as close to your head as possible. Push right back and return to your starting position.

Major muscles involved:
There are many muscles at work here. Clavicular pectoralis muscles (upper chest) are involved, although you may not really feel them a lot. The triceps brachii (back of arm) is doing a tremendous amount of work at the pushing-up motion, and it is the prime mover in this exercise. The pushing-up motion forces the rectus abdominis to stabilize your core and, thus, a great amount of force is generated through that muscle. Another stabilizing muscle

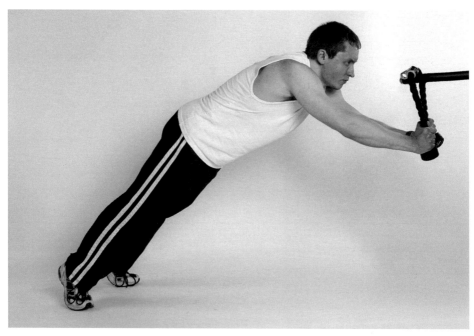

Photo 1.38

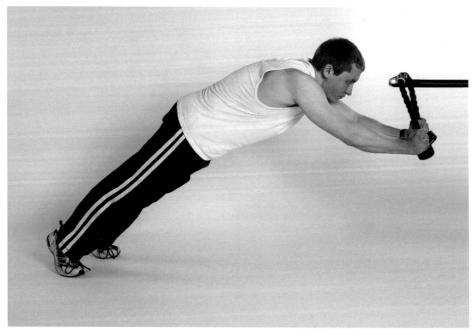

Photo 1.39

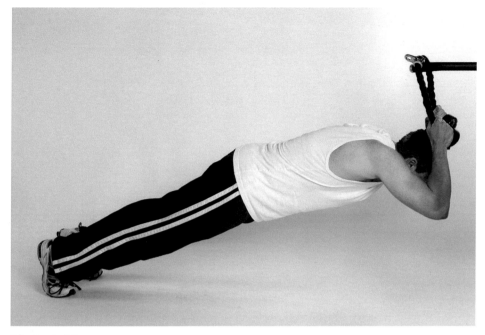

Photo 1.40

in the Hanuman Extension is latissimus dorsi (side of back). Serratus anterior is also part of the stabilizing muscle group in this exercise.

Ark's tips:
Make sure you go slow and meditate on the tension of muscles in the arms and core. Remember, the closer you keep the elbows to the head, the more you isolate your triceps.

Breathing technique:
Inhale as you go down and exhale as you commence to push yourself up. You can momentarily hold your breath at the hardest point of the exercise, which is the very moment you start pushing back up.

Sports applications:
Hanuman Extension will benefit martial artists who break boards or objects using a sword hand swing as it specifically strengthens the core and triceps in the downward phase of the sword hand strike. It will benefit gymnasts balancing on a bar or a pummel horse due to its tremendous stress on the gripping power and back-of-arm strength. It will also aid athletes whose sport discipline involves pushing, such as boxing, martial arts (various punches), and football (linemen pushing, hitting, repelling). Hanuman Extensions may prove beneficial to volleyball athletes who jump high to spike and/or block the ball.

Come on, warrior, you're not done yet!/progression:

IDP2:
Lift one foot up and perform the exercise.

    Bhishmadeva's Running Wild Row

    Difficulty level: I

    Origin: ID

    Presenter: Warrior Marcin

Starting position:
Attach a bar to an adjustable pulley. The pulley should align with your chest or be slightly lower when you squat. Adjust your weight. Get in a partial lunge position by moving the right leg back. Take the bar in your hands in a palm-down fashion; bend your knees (see Photo 1.41).

Movement:
Contract abdominals and the lower back. While holding the bar, take at least three quick steps back. Stop in a lunge position and perform two rowing motions with the bar by pulling the bar close to your chest and back (see Photos 1.42–46). Next, run back to the pulley and then return for another two rows. Perform 10 runs of two rows in this fashion.

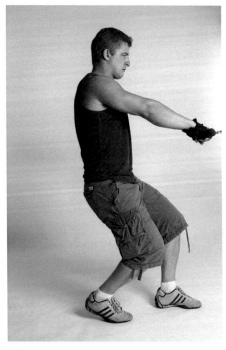

Photo 1.41

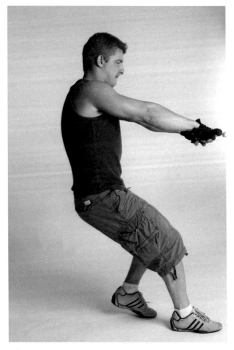

Photo 1.42

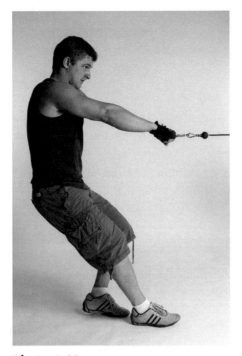

Photo 1.43

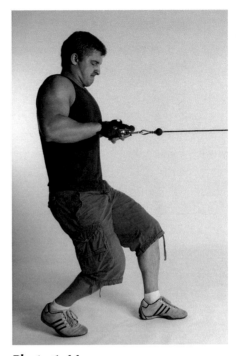

Photo 1.44

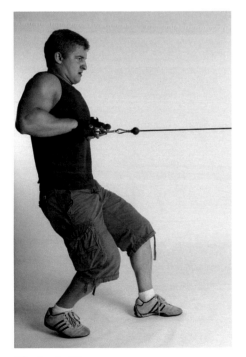

Photo 1.45

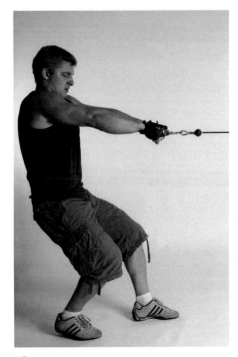

Photo 1.46

Major muscles involved:

The main muscle at work is the latissimus dorsi, the side of your back. The muscles of the core stabilize your torso while you run and pull the weight. Also, because you are in a partial lunge position, your leg muscles will do some work.

Ark's tips:

Do not make it a "lazy walk." Run! But make sure you first see that there is nothing behind you that you could run into. Inhale when rowing in and exhale when rowing out. Keep your core straight along the center line of your body. In other words, your upper body should be perpendicular to the floor. Keep your head up. When you run forward, obviously, the weight of the pulley will push you forward, so it is good to judge the force of the pull and oppose the resistance. This will also engage the muscles of the core. Then when you run back, resistance will change direction.

Breathing technique:

When running, perform quick inhalations and exhalations from your lower abdominals (karate breathing) and longer ones when rowing.

Sports applications:

This is excellent for any sport that involves rowing. Also gymnasts, tennis, and badminton players will benefit from this exercise. As an example from tennis, we may give the execution of the backhand. Running backward will strengthen leg muscles for some short duration, high nonlinear anaerobic activities, such as footwork in soccer or basketball.

Come on, warrior, you're not done yet!/progression:

IDP1:

Lift your back foot when rowing.

> Karate Squats
>
> Difficulty level: I
>
> Caution: If you have back or knee problems, you may be able to perform the exercise modification provided.
>
> Origin: K
>
> Presenter: Warrior Rich

Starting position:

Squat all the way down so that you are in a crouching position (your calf and back of thigh will touch), resting on the balls of your feet with your hands supporting your body in front of the feet (see Photo 1.47).

Movement:

While keeping hands touching the floor, straighten out your legs as much as you can without taking your hands off the floor (see Photos 1.48–51). You will most likely feel a pull in the

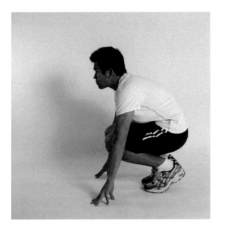

Photo 1.47

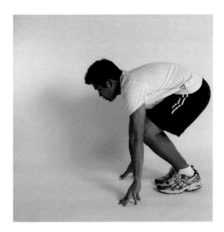

Photo 1.48

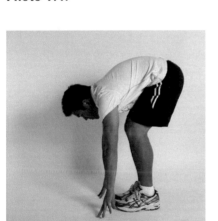

Photo 1.49

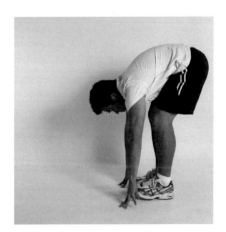

Photo 1.50

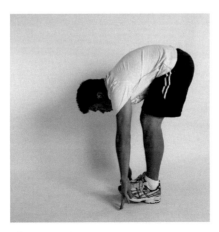

Photo 1.51

hamstrings (back of thigh), which means that you are stretching those particular muscles and tendons. Then return to a starting position. Repeat 15 times.

Major muscles involved:
In this exercise, there is a lot of quadriceps work involved, such as vastus medialis and lateralis. To a minor degree, calf muscles (especially gastrocnemius) are at work here.

Ark's tips:
If you are not a martial artist or practice a sport that involves extending your leg in a fast manner (like kicking or sprinting), you can, for general flexibility purposes, do the Karate Squat slowly, even with holding at the end (when legs are straight). Otherwise, you should do the exercise somewhat fast to make it a more specific muscle movement and a dynamic stretch.

Breathing technique:
Exhale going up and inhale going down.

Sports applications:
Combative art practitioners will benefit from Karate Squats a great deal, and especially those involving kicking. Knee extension exercises benefit especially jumpers, runners, martial artists who kick, power lifters, football players, etc. They are useful in developing basic skills in those sports. The gastrocnemius in the calf will help in such essential motor skills as walking, running, and jumping.

Come on, warrior, you're not done yet!/progression:

IDP1:
After extending your legs out, hold the stretch phase of the exercise for 5 seconds.

Modification (for flexion-biased persons[8] and/or for persons with knee problems):
Perform a simple reverse lunge; that is, step back with one foot until both knees are bent at 90 degrees or less (the angle measured between the calf and back of the thigh). Make sure that back foot is resting on its ball and the heel is pointing straight up. Return to your starting position and step back with the other leg.

Okay, now, let's repeat this sequence twice more and then check our stopwatch for the time completed, and then we can proceed to a cooldown.

Cooldown. Walk around for a minute and perform stretches for the muscles worked during the training session,[9] such as front shoulders, chest, triceps (back of arm), etc.

Ending meditation:
Perform steps 1 and 2 in the beginning meditation.

Draw the outstretched hands to the sides of your chest in the same manner as you did at the beginning of the session. Then simply open your hands so the palms are facing down and gradually and smoothly release your air as you lower your hands to your hips. At this time, you are absorbing rejuvenating energy from the body of the Supreme Warrior and allowing it to return to the center of your energy (the energy point below the navel). With gratitude and surrender, accept this energy from the Supreme Lord. Repeat the breathing sequence until you feel calm, joyful, and energetic.

Return hands to the position from step 1.

Slowly stand up.

Word of instruction:

Congratulations! You have completed the first workout plan. Just stay focused on the mission, warrior! Continue with the workout for the next 6 weeks, three times a week, each time trying to better your form and take less rest. As you train, write down your completion times on your Personal Record Sheet (see Chapter 5). On other days, engage yourself in jogging, sports of your liking, or skill training that you may need for your specific discipline (football or soccer practice, performing kata, or forms in karate). Try to eat in accordance with your body type 7 days a week. Make sure to take 1 day of complete rest.

FINAL ASSIGNMENTS

1. (Required) At the end of the sixth week, perform a fitness assessment on yourself or have someone do it for you. See how much fat weight you've lost and how many pounds of lean muscle you've gained.

2. (Required) If you gained muscle and lost body fat, you will need to increase your protein intake to keep making gains (increase strength, power, etc.) and burn more fat. If you are a competitive athlete, you should apply protein recommendations that your body type requires (see Chapter 4), as well as necessary supplements (e.g., L-carnitine, creatine monohydrate, etc.).

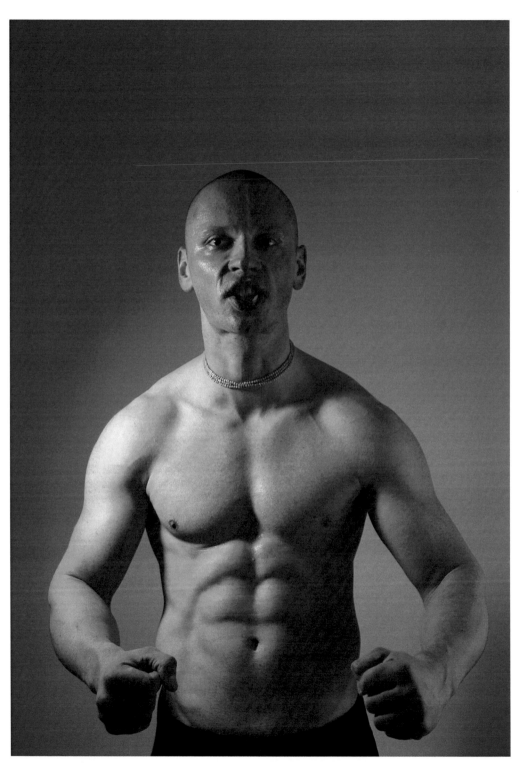

Come on, let's go!

Chapter II

Intermediate Krishna Warrior Program

THE CASTLE OF MIND

"Every endeavor is covered by some fault, just as fire is covered by smoke. But one should not give up the work born of his nature . . . even if such work is faulty."

Bhagavad-Gita 18.48

"Who is there?" I asked loudly from behind the altar, although I knew who was training next.

"Goru! It's me, Ark!" The boy walked in, paid his respects to Narasimhadeva and Master Orayen, and came up to me.

I did not say anything for a moment and waited.

"You know, Ark, I don't feel like I should do the training today . . . I feel sluggish and tired and—"

"You don't feel the power today, do you?" I asked and looked at Narasimhadeva.

"Not even a bit . . ." Goru hung his head down.

"You've got finals, don't you?" I asked and took out a bottle of peppermint oil.

"Yeah, I've been studying all night and got only two or three hours of sleep. I don't want to waste your time . . . It won't be productive. I know you will push me, but today just isn't the right day."

I laughed. "Look at him! Goru, the warrior, is speaking like that. You wanted to be a powerful man, but sometimes it's not so easy, right? Disciplining yourself is hard sometimes, right?" I grabbed his hand and poured a few drops of peppermint oil on it.

"Sniff it, boy. The fight is not over yet." I made him look into my eyes. "Deep inside, you really want to give up because you think you can't handle it today. But you don't want to let me down or upset me, and that's why you still made it to the door to tell me this, right?"

"Yeah. I did not want to call you on the phone. I wanted you to know that I care." Goru sniffed the strong oil a few times.

"You don't want to upset me, but you don't care for your workout today. Otherwise, you would do it anyway." I looked at him fiercely.

"Yeah, but . . ." Goru was feeling the challenge I was posing.

"But that is why you have Narasimhadeva and me to give you the power when you are really desperate."

Goru looked at me and then looked longer at Lord Narasimhadeva. He was meditating. Then he looked at me, and I placed his hand with peppermint oil under his nose again.

"Ten times, boy, 10 times." I took out my stopwatch.

"Why 10 times, man?" Goru looked frustrated.

"'Cause that's what it says in the book. Listen, let's do it. The sense of accomplishment will come later. Do not expect everything to be perfect but intend to do your best and perform your duty externally. Don't do this for yourself or even me . . . Do it for—"

"—the Supreme Warrior, Krishna!" finished Goru and started running around the gym making arm circles.

I looked at Lord Narasimhadeva and Master Prabhupada and then at Goru. Goru's One-armed Push-ups were terrible, but when I saw his face twisted in pain and determination, I did not correct him. "Good effort, Goru. Good effort. Make sure to eat light when you get home and go to sleep early tonight."

SILVER DOOR 2: THE CASTLE OF INTELLIGENCE

REQUIRED ASSIGNMENTS

Now that you have passed through the first phase of training your body, mind, and spirit, you are ready to further commit yourself to the rigorous and rewarding lifestyle of a Krishna warrior.

All serious Krishna warriors recite the following oath in the morning:

1. I will forge my mind and body in the fire of spiritual and physical discipline, as set by previous self-realized masters (e.g., Arjuna, Bhishmadeva, Buddha, etc.).
2. I will faithfully exercise my body in this spirit so that in time, by the Supreme Warrior's will, I will come to the point of pure love for all men and God.
3. Above all, I pledge to dedicate the results, or any benefits derived, from physical exercise, as well as the training itself, to the Supreme Warrior Krishna (God), who is the greatest warrior. All power and strength come from him.
4. I will not use my skills frivolously but only in accordance with a definite plan from my trainer/superior.
5. To become successful in this endeavor, I will shield myself with the armor of surrender and the power of the Lord's holy name, knowing that They are the source of my power, so help me, Lord.

BRONZE DOOR 2

ASSIGNMENTS:

1. (Required) If you have not already done so, adjust your food intake according to your body composition change.
2. (Required) Continue your cleansing phase by going to the next level. To do that, follow your body type diet, refrain from all flesh food, and refrain from eating grains (any breads, cakes, cookies, noodles, cereals) and beans twice a month (for acid reduction).

If you are not prepared to do that, then do not consume flesh food twice a month (on days when you abstain from grains and beans). For the rest of the month, consume flesh only once a day, around noon (when digestive acid is very strong). Consume more vegetables and fruits. Use lemon essential oil with any water you drink.

3. (Required) Fill out your Personal Achievement Goal Sheet (PAG) for the second month (see Chapter 5). Continue with the Transcendental Warrior Achievement Program as described in the first chapter.

4. (Optional) If needed, modify your daily schedule with, most importantly, workout times and workout types included.

5. (Optional) Continue filling out your Personal Record Sheet (PRS) (see Chapter 5).

GOLDEN DOOR 2: MEDITATION

Use the same meditation as in the Beginner's KWFC plan.

Warm-up. Duration of about 5 minutes.

Equipment needed: None

Presenter: Warrior Susan

Execution:

Push-up position, push-up (not shown), crouching position, kick legs out in a push-up position, back to crouching position, explode up, land in crouching position, push-up position, push-up (see Photos 2X.1–8). Repeat at least 15 times.

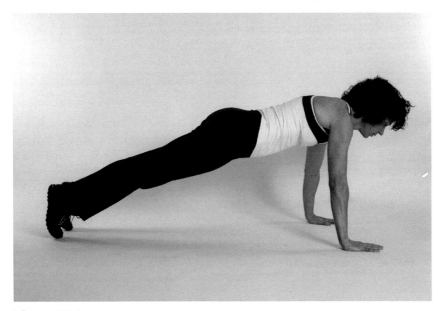

Photo 2X.1

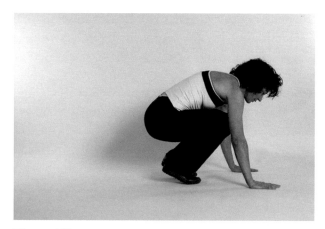

Photo 2X.2

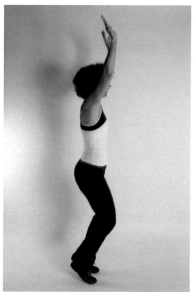

Photo 2X.5

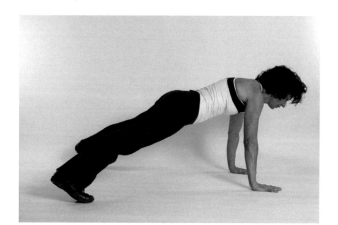

Photo 2X.3

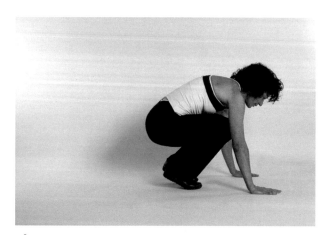

Photo 2X.4

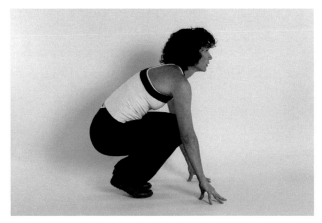

Photo 2X.6

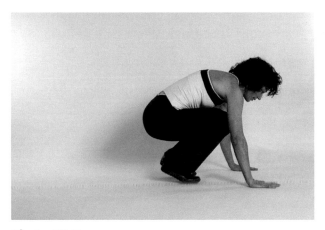

Photo 2X.7

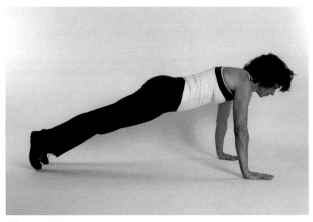

Photo 2X.8

Comments: Keep the core (abdominals, lower back) and thighs tight when performing push-ups and kicking legs out to be in a push-up position.

Equipment needed: Floor, mat, elastic band, adjustable pulley station

Progression: Add more push-ups and more explosions to the sequence.

EXERCISES IN THE MAIN CORE OF THE WORKOUT

Equipment needed: Adjustable pulley stations, mat, elastic bands, two pair of light dumbbells (between 5 and 10 pounds), incline bench, medicine ball (or plate), stopwatch.

Estimated Completion Time: 45 minutes

General Comments: ECT listed above was calculated during a rather medium-paced workout. Time to quickly adjust pulleys and bands is included. Meditation and warm-up times are not included. If you go over 45 minutes, then you probably rested too long between exercises and/or sequences. Remember, the idea behind the PHA system of training is to go NONSTOP. For a competitive finishing time of the intermediate workout with my own loading parameters, see Chapter 5, Physical Assessments.

SEQUENCE 1 (REPEATED THREE TIMES IN A CIRCUITLIKE FASHION):
   Nakula's J Cross
   Tiger Push-ups
   Dragon Fly
   Krishna Warrior Biceps Curl
   Karna's Fall

SEQUENCE 2 (REPEATED THREE TIMES IN A CIRCUITLIKE FASHION):
   Low Pulley Uppercuts
   Kung Fu Triceps Extension
   Asvatthama's Row
   Master Crunch
   Crouching Tiger

SEQUENCE 3 (REPEATED THREE TIMES IN A CIRCUITLIKE FASHION):

Flying Eagle

Parasurama's Power Punch

Eccentric Sit-up with Medicine Ball

Balarama's Squats

DESCRIPTIONS OF EXERCISES IN THE INTERMEDIATE PROGRAM, SEQUENCE 1

Nakula's J Cross

Difficulty level: I

Origin: ID

Presenter: Warrior Kim D.

Starting position:
Stand in a neutral position holding two lightweight dumbbells (start with 3, 4, or 5 pounds) in front of you. Hold the dumbbells in a palm-down position. See Photo 2.1.

Movement:
Commence by raising both dumbbells all the way until your arms are over your head (see Photo 2.2) or perpendicular to the floor and, without stopping, in a smooth motion, lower them to the side (see Photo 2.3). As you bring your arms down, your hands will be in a neutral, palm-forward position. Lower them halfway so that your arms end up at a shoulder height level. Then bring them up again and down along the same path to the starting position. Repeat and continue in the same fashion for 12 times.

Major muscles involved:
In the first phase of the movement (raising of dumbbells), the anterior deltoid (front shoulder) muscle is involved. In the lowering of the dumbbells, the medial deltoid (outer shoulder) muscle acts as the prime mover and the posterior deltoid (rear shoulder) acts as the assisting mover. The anterior deltoid works again in bringing dumbbells along the horizontal plane to a starting position.

Ark's tips:
Keep your arms straight with a slight bend in the elbow joint. Make a smooth transition between the raising up and lowering of the dumbbells. Do not use heavy dumbbells for this exercise.

Breathing technique:
Exhale going up and inhale going down. Then exhale again when your arms travel from your sides to the front (along a horizontal plane). Pause for a second while inhaling and raise the dumbbells up again while you exhale.

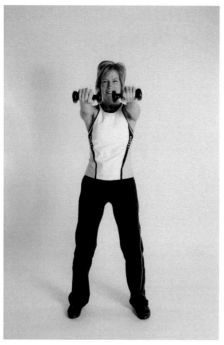

Photo 2.1

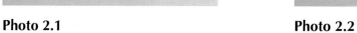

Photo 2.2

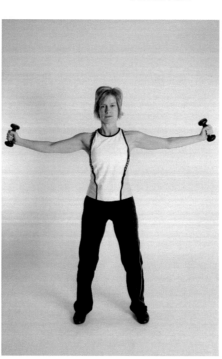

Photo 2.3

Sports applications:

The raising up phase of the movement is particularly useful in gymnastics, diving, basketball, and volleyball (e.g., when you reach up to block the ball). A strong front shoulder is also needed in boxing to get the arm up (e.g., keeping hands on guard) or in the uppercut. It is also needed in judo and wrestling. The lowering portion of the movement works the outer shoulder and is also beneficial in volleyball, basketball (e.g., blocking, guarding stance), and tennis (e.g., serving). The lowering portion of the J Cross also works your rear shoulder, and thus helps in sports that involve rowing, tennis (backhand), and archery (pulling the string back).

Come on, warrior, you're not done yet!/progression:

IDP1:

While bringing the dumbbells up to a vertical position, stop the movement right in the middle and pause for 5 seconds. Resume the movement all the way up. As you lower the dumbbells out to the sides, pause again for 5 seconds right in the middle of going down. Resume movement until your arms are stretched out and aligned with your shoulders. When you bring them back up to a vertical position, pause again halfway and complete the movement. Start going down to a horizontal position and pause halfway for 5 seconds. Complete the movement until the arms are aligned with your shoulders and parallel to the floor (horizontal).

Tiger Push-ups

Difficulty level: A

Origin: K

Presenter: Warrior Greg

Starting position:

Begin by getting into a regular push-up position, that is, supporting yourself on the palms of your hands and two feet. Your feet can be spread at shoulder width, with arms and fingers pointing forward, placed on the mat approximately shoulder width apart or a little wider (see Photo 2.4).

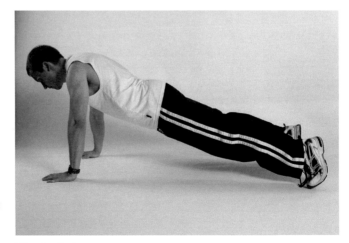

Photo 2.4

Movement:

Inhale, draw your abdominals in, shift your whole body back starting with your forearms so that your hips come up high and your shoulders are behind in relation to your hands (see Photo 2.5). Next, dive down so that you land on the elbows (forearms), with your chest almost touching the floor (keep your elbows in, touching the sides). See Photo 2.6. Your hips are still up in the air, and your shoulders (and chest) are still behind in relation to your hands. Then, contracting the muscles of the core maximally, push yourself forward (so your chest brushes your hands) and up until you end up in a cobra position (push-up position but with hips down). See Photo 2.7. Adjust your hips up so that you are in a regular push-up position and repeat 14 more times.

Major muscles involved:

There are many muscles at work here. Clavicular pectoralis muscles (upper chest) are involved, although you may not really feel them a lot. The triceps brachii (back of arm) is doing a tremendous amount of work at the pushing-up motion, and it is the prime mover in this exercise. The anterior deltoid (front shoulder) muscle is assisting the pectoralis and triceps brachii muscles in the pushing motion. The pushing-up motion forces the rectus abdominis to stabilize your core and, thus, a great amount of force is generated through that muscle. Another stabilizing muscle in Tiger Push-ups is latissimus dorsi (side of back). Serratus anterior is also part of the stabilizing muscle group in Tiger Push-ups.

Ark's tips:

Make the movement smooth. The slower the exercise is performed, the harder it gets. For explosive athletes, you may want to do it faster and do more repetitions. For strength athletes, you should do Tiger Push-ups slower but with fewer repetitions. Keeping the elbows close in and moving close to the floor ensures the right amount of stress to the muscles. If you can't get it right, it is better to try Tiger Push-ups on your knees and not cheat on the original exercise. Push from the bottom outer ends of your palms.

Breathing technique:

Inhale as you shift your body backward and begin exhaling as you dive down to the floor. The final exhalation should occur during the pushing-up motion when you straighten out your hands.

Sports applications:

Tiger Push-ups will benefit anybody whose sport discipline involves pushing, such as boxing (jab), martial arts (various punches),[10] football (linemen pushing, hitting, repelling), discus throwing, etc.

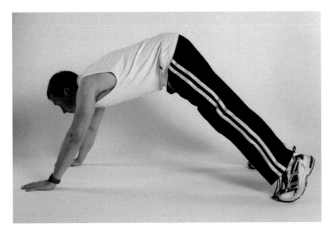

Photo 2.5

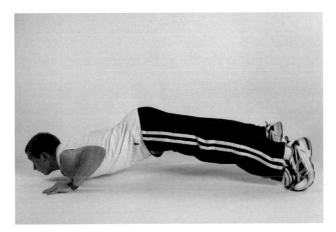

Photo 2.6

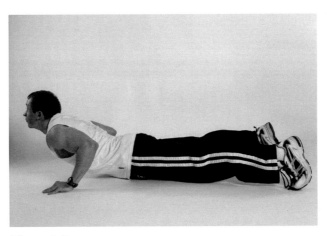

Photo 2.7

Come on, warrior, you're not done yet!/progression:

IDP1:

Rest on your knees and place one hand behind your back. Perform the same movement.

> Dragon Fly
>
> Caution: If you have back problems, you may be able to perform the exercise modification provided.
>
> Difficulty level: I
>
> Origin: ID
>
> Presenter: Self

Starting position:

Attach an elastic band to a low pulley so the band is fastened just above the floor. Sit up on a mat with your feet toward the low pulley. Grab the two handles of the band, one with each hand (see Photo 2.8).

Movement:

Tighten up your abdominal muscles and while extending the two elastic bands to the side and up, rock back from the sitting up position until your shoulder blades touch the floor (see Photos 2.9–2.11). The arms should travel above your shoulders. Your legs should be up in the air and slightly bent. As you commence the return phase of the movement, maintain a stable contracted core, bring your arms down to your sides, and rock your way back up to a sitting position. Perform 15 Dragon Flies.

Major muscles involved:

Rectus abdominis, along with transverse abdominis and oblique muscles, stabilizes the core while medial deltoid (outer shoulder) moves the arms up against resistance created by the band.

Ark's tips:

The straighter you keep your legs, the harder it will be for you to generate kinetic momentum and overcome resistance created by the band. It will also be harder on the abs to stabilize your trunk. Keep your arms almost straight to increase stress on the medial deltoid. You may help yourself by pushing off with your heels at the commencement of each repetition. Try to

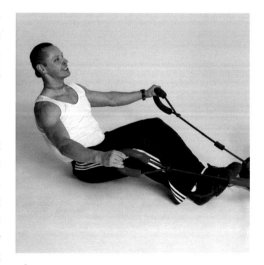

Photo 2.8

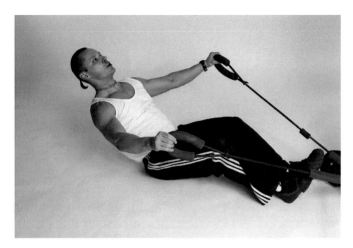

Photo 2.9

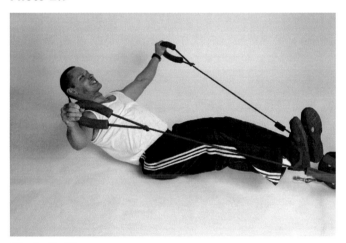

Photo 2.10

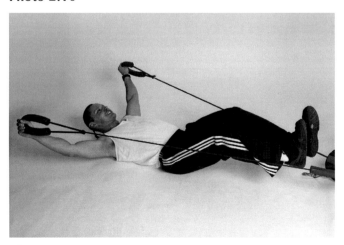

Photo 2.11

minimize the time when your shoulder blades or heels touch the floor. This exercise utilizes very similar body mechanics to those in the Rocking Chair exercise described in the beginner's program.

Breathing technique:
Exhale rocking back and inhale coming back to a sitting position.

Sports applications:
This exercise can help athletes in disciplines such as basketball, baseball, or football. In basketball, the player often jumps in the air (abdominal action), twists the torso at the same time, and shoots or blocks the ball (outer shoulder and abdominal action). The core is often partially contracted in such air battles, and the transverse abdominis muscle is used in sports with short-term power activities; it pulls abs inward, forcing exhalation. In baseball, the action of the outer shoulder is crucial in catching overhead flies. In football, arms go overhead during various tackles. Practitioners of martial arts such as karate will also derive benefit from the Dragon Fly by strengthening the core in a dynamic way as well as shoulders. In karate, for example, there is a strike called *uraken saio uchi* (pronounced "saeyo") that utilizes the action of the outer shoulder in a very fast way.

Come on, warrior, you're not done yet!/progression:
Once you complete the movement with your arms, hold them extended out for a second or two while breaking with one of your legs. Break by bending and putting the heel of one foot down. Then let go and start another repetition. You will not have the same dynamic momentum in this modified version of Dragon Fly. However, you will tax your shoulders and hamstrings pretty hard because of the pausing and holding element (isometric contractions).

Modification (for extension-biased persons[11]):
Lie on the mat with knees bent. Make sure the small of your back touches the floor. Perform a horizontal shoulder raise with two elastic bands.

Krishna Warrior Biceps Curl

Difficulty level: I

Origin: ID

Presenter: Warrior Kim D.

Starting position:
Spread out a mat next to a pulley station. Adjust the cable pulley to a high position (a few notches down, though) and attach a handle to it. Set on a low weight (between 25 and 40 pounds). Holding the handle with the right hand, lie down on the mat with legs bent and face the pulley stand. Extend your right leg out into the air so it is aligned with your extended right arm holding the handle. Extend the left arm out to the side so the back of your shoulder does not touch the mat. Keep your chin down. Next, push down with the heel of the left foot into

the floor, thus, lifting the small of your back from the mat. Your right leg and torso should form one straight line. The only points of contact with the mat are upper back and heel (see Photo 2.12).

Movement:
While holding the above described position, perform 15 curling motions with the right arm. See Photos 2.13–2.14. Switch arms and legs.

Major muscles involved:
Quite a few of them are involved here! Let's start with the prime mover, which is the biceps brachii (front of arm). Biceps femoris (back of thigh/hamstring), gluteus maximus (buttock), and erector spinae (lower back) are the three main stabilizing muscles in the Krishna Warrior Curl. Other muscles in use are rectus abdominis (abdominals), external oblique (sides), as well as posterior deltoid (back shoulder).

Ark's tips:
The key to performing this Krishna Warrior Curl is holding the position right. Make sure your core is stable (tight) after you push the hip as high as you can (it won't be easy, of course). The challenge of the exercise lies in the awkward position you're in. Use a medium to slow tempo when doing curls. The longer you stay in the position, the better.

Breathing technique:
Exhale as you curl and inhale as you extend your arm.

Sports applications:
The Krishna Warrior Biceps Curl is great for strengthening your lower back muscles, back of legs, and butt. It will help in all sports that require rising up with an arched back. We may mention weight lifting (power cleans, squat, dead lift), baseball (fielding, catching overhead balls), football (linemen coming off the line), as well as jumping activities of basketball (jumping for rebounds). Often in sports such as basketball or volleyball, an athlete will assume a hyperextended position in the air, as in spiking, for example.

Come on, warrior, you're not done yet!/progression:

IDP1:
Hold a 10- to 25-pound plate in your extended arm and perform the KW Curl with the added weight.

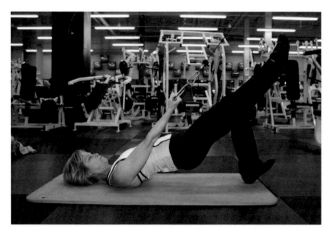

Photo 2.12

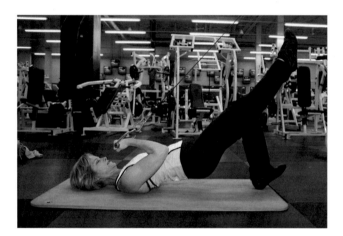

Photo 2.13

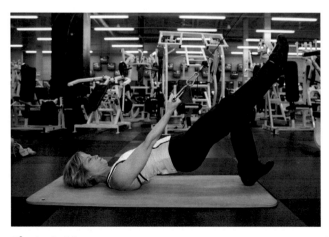

Photo 2.14

Karna's Fall/Defense Fall and Get Up

Difficulty level: A

Caution: If you have knee problems, you may be able to perform the exercise modification provided.

Origin: K

Presenter: Self

Starting position:

Place a mat behind you. Assume a shoulder width foot stance. Slightly bend at the hips, knees, and arms (a 90-degree angle or so). See Photo 2.15.

Movement:

Commence the exercise by rapidly squatting down and, while cushioning yourself with the palms of your hands (especially if you do not have a soft mat), falling onto the mat (see Photos 2.16–18). Keep your chin down and tighten your abdominal muscles. Once on the mat, keep falling backward until your shoul-

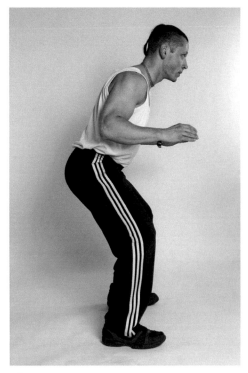

Photo 2.15

der blades touch the mat and your legs are up (see Photo 2.19). All the while, your arms are positioned on the mat to your sides. They are cushioning and controlling the movement. When you start losing kinetic momentum generated from the fall, tighten the abdominals even more, push off with your hands, and jerk your legs forward as you crunch up (see Photo 2.20).

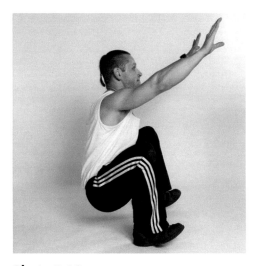

Photo 2.16

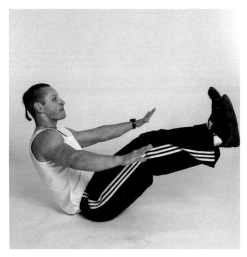

Photo 2.17

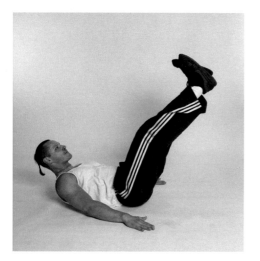

Photo 2.18

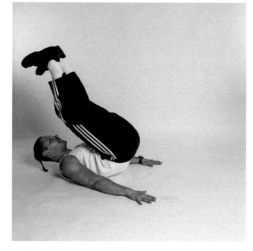

Photo 2.19

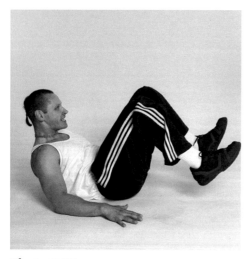

Photo 2.20

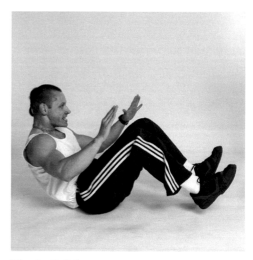

Photo 2.21

Your shoulder blades will come off the mat, and you are rolling forward (see Photos 2.21–22). Bend the legs quickly so that your calves and the back of the thighs (hamstrings) touch. See Photo 2.23. You should stand up as soon as your tailbone comes off the mat and return to the initial squatting position. Perform 15 Karna Falls.

Major muscles involved:
The muscles here work in the same way as in squatting. As you flex your knee, the rectus femoris (front of thigh) does the majority of the work. Assisting in the movement are: biceps femoris (back of thigh) and gluteus maximus (butt). The erector spinae (lower back), rectus

abdominis, as well as external oblique muscles contract isometrically to stabilize the torso. As you fall back and start rolling, your rectus abdominis continues to work.

Ark's tips:
You have to make the movement dynamic enough to be able to get yourself back up on your feet. In addition, you should use your hands to push off at the right time. As you are on your way rocking back, keep your arms and especially your forearms on the mat so that you are using them to gradually push yourself up. When your heels are already touching the mat (but the whole foot is still pointing up), you perform the final push-off with your hands.

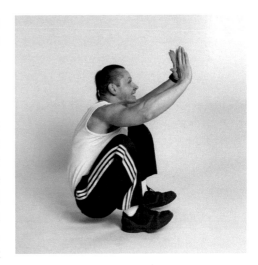

Photo 2.22

Breathing technique:
Breathe in when falling down and start exhaling on your way back up. The final exhaling phase (at which you may hold your breath for a split second) should occur when your butt is off the mat and you are squatting up from a very low position (less than a 90-degree angle between the back of your thigh and calf). Exhale forcefully the rest of the air. Tighten up those stomach muscles.

Sports applications:
This is essentially a defense fall, so it will greatly help various martial arts practitioners who may be covering this kind of defensive behavior in their training program. The explosive form of a squat will help athletes who perform many jumping actions, such as volleyball and basketball players in their air battles.

Come on, warrior, you're not done yet!/progression:

IDP1:
Do not use hands in the last phase of going up (see the picture). This will force you to be more dynamic and tax your leg muscles more.

IDP2:
Once you get up from the mat, jump into the air and perform a 180-degree turn. You should end up in the same squatting position (it can be slightly wider). Using the kinetic momentum from the jump, quickly reload and in a split second, jump back in reverse direction (also 180 degrees). Then proceed with your next fall and get up in the manner described above.

IDP3:
Try holding a plate close to your chest, and as you complete standing up from a squat position, lift the plate overhead or in front of you.

Modification (for persons with knee conditions):
Perform a simple partial squat, that is, bend your knees so that the angle between the back of your thigh and calf is approximately 135 degrees.

Great, now let's repeat this sequence twice more before we move on to sequence 2!

DESCRIPTIONS OF EXERCISES IN THE INTERMEDIATE PROGRAM, SEQUENCE 2

Low Pulley Uppercuts

Difficulty level: B

Origin: IDP

Presenter: Warrior Bill

Starting position:
Set two adjustable pulleys at the lowest point and attach two handles to them. Adjust the weight to your strength. Stand between the pulleys, grab two handles, and place your palms at your sides. Keep your knees slightly bent (see Photo 2.23).

Movement:
The Curl is very similar to a regular Biceps Curl, except that it should be a little exaggerated and faster. You are using the whole body to curl the weight up. As you turn your torso to the left, turn your right foot in the same direction and start curling with the right hand (see Photo 2.24). As you commence the movement, your right hand is turning up so that

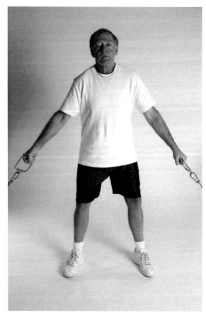

Photo 2.23

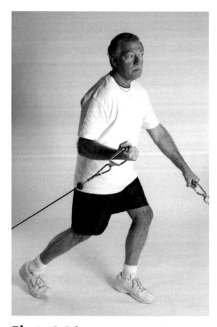

Photo 2.24

you end up with your flexed palm facing up (see Photo 2.25). You are almost facing the left pulley. As you return with your right foot, start turning and curling with left arm (see Photos 2.26–28). The two movements kind of blend into each other; that is, you don't wait

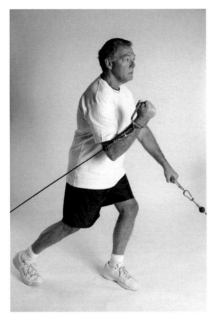

Photo 2.25

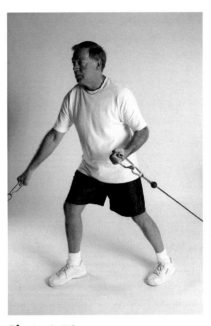

Photo 2.26

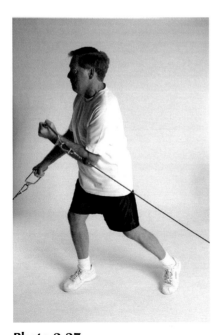

Photo 2.27

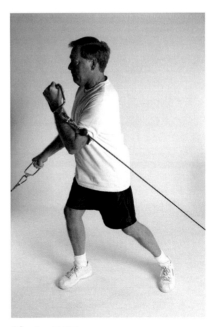

Photo 2.28

until the completion of the right Curl before starting the left Curl. It is very similar to uppercuts in boxing or karate. Uppercut 15 times with each arm.

Major muscles involved:
Major muscles at work are: biceps brachii (front of arm) and external oblique (sides). Assisting muscles are: serratus anterior (ribcage muscles) and anterior deltoid (front of your shoulder).

Ark's tips:
Make the movement smooth. Shift your weight from one foot to the other as you curl. To be more specific, start shifting your weight from one foot to the other even before you start curling. For example, if you intend to curl with the right arm, begin shifting weight from the right to the left leg a split second before you start curling.

Breathing technique:
Breathe out as you curl up and breathe in at the moment when you complete the curl on one arm and before you curl with the other arm (there is a split-second pause at that time).

Sports applications:
Almost any martial arts practitioner will derive benefit from this combat-specific movement. Disciplines like kickboxing, boxing, karate, judo, and wrestling should have this exercise included in their combat drills (using weights, cables, or bands). For example, in judo, which is the art of unbalancing your opponent and throwing him to the ground, Low Pulley Uppercuts will assist the action of grabbing and pulling in an opponent from an outreached position. In wrestling, you also need to pull an opponent into position before you throw him.

Come on, warrior, you're not done yet!/progression:

IDP2:
As you are about to complete a right uppercut, lift the right leg by bending it to about a 90-degree angle. Complete the uppercut in this unstable position.

> Kung Fu Triceps Extension/High Pulley Single Arm-leg Triceps Extension
>
> Difficulty level: I
>
> Origin: ID
>
> Presenter: Warrior Kim D.

Starting position:
Adjust the pulley station to at least a head level and attach a handle to it. Set a light weight, grab the handle with your right hand, and turn your back to the station. Thus, facing away from the pulley station, lift your left knee up and extend your left arm out to the side. Then, raise your right elbow so it is almost parallel to the floor. See Photo 2.29.

Movement:
Perform 15 right arm extensions as shown in Photos 2.30–31. Switch arms and legs.

Major muscles involved:
Triceps brachii (back of arm) is the prime mover in the Kung Fu Extension. Anterior deltoid (front shoulder) is stabilizing the arm in the parallel-to-floor position. Core muscles (abdominals, obliques), as well as back extensors (lower back), are stabilizing the trunk to make the upper body motion possible. Gluteus maximus (buttock) is the stabilizing muscle for the lower body (of the leg you are standing on).

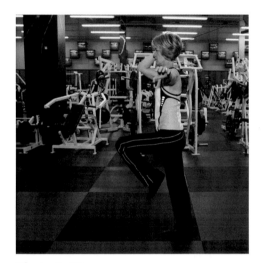

Photo 2.29

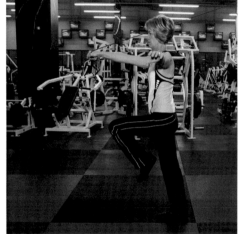

Photo 2.30

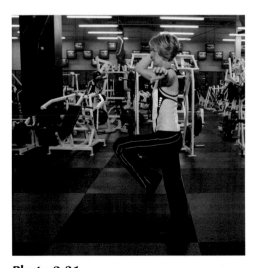

Photo 2.31

Ark's tips:
Keep the right arm close to your side and try not to move the upper arm (everything from elbow up). In this way, you will involve the triceps brachii more. Keep the core muscles and your buttock (of the leg you are standing on) very tight so that you do not lose balance. Do not lower your left knee.

Breathing technique:
Inhale as you extend the arm and exhale as you flex it.

Sports applications:
This exercise is specific to sports like volleyball (jumping up to spike or even block) or badminton since it involves isometric contraction of core muscles while extending the arm. Kung Fu Extension will benefit martial artists who break boards or objects using a sword hand swing as it specifically strengthens the core and triceps in the initial phase of the sword hand strike.

Come on, warrior, you're not done yet!/progression:

IDP1:
Begin from the starting position described above but hold a light dumbbell in the free hand and/or perform a left hip flexion simultaneously with right arm extension.

    Asvatthama's Row/Dynamic Alternated Row with Lunge on High Pulley

    Difficulty level: I

    Origin: IDP

    Presenter: Warrior Kim D.

Starting position:
Adjust the pulley so that it is above your head. Attach a handle and set a weight that is not overly heavy for pulling with a single arm (65–70 percent of what you can maximally lift). Face the pulley, hold the handle by a neutral grip in the left hand and step back with your left foot (partial right lead lunge position). Pull your left arm holding the handle toward you until it is almost chest high (and close to your chest). See Photo 2.32.

Movement:
Suddenly move your left leg to where your right leg is resting. Almost instantaneously, take your

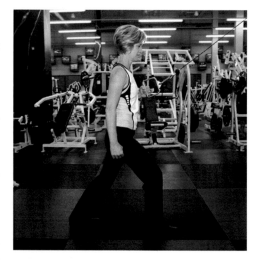

Photo 2.32

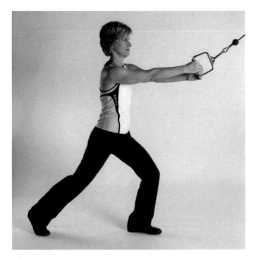

Photo 2.33

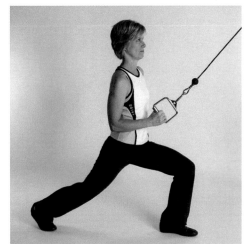

Photo 2.34

right leg back, switch grips (see Photo 2.33), and pull your right hand now, holding the pulley toward you.

You should end up in a left lead lunge position (left leg bent at a 90-degree angle with foot flat and right leg partially bent with the ball of your right foot resting on the floor) with your right hand close to your side and almost chest high (see Photo 2.34). This is opposite of your starting position.

With the same speed, move your right foot forward to where your left foot was resting. Your right arm should simultaneously travel forward and up and release the tension of the pulley. When your feet are on their way to being separated again, instantaneously switch grips on the handle and lunge back with the left foot while pulling the handle with your left hand. This brings you back to your starting position and counts as one repetition. Repeat 10 times in the same manner.

Major muscles involved:

We've got quite a few muscles involved here. In fact, the whole body! Let's list some major ones. First of all, the rowing motion involves latissimus dorsi (side of back), which serves as the prime mover of the upper body in this exercise. Assisting the latissimus are biceps brachii (front arm) and posterior deltoid (rear shoulder). In the lower body, we have the whole quadriceps group (rectus femoris, vastus medialis, vastus lateralis, sartorius), as well as the hamstring group (biceps femoris, semitendinosus, semimembranosus). Of course, the calves and lower extremities are involved in the balance function of the entire body. Muscles of the core are engaged in the process of stabilizing, while those of the upper and lower body execute specific movements.

Ark's tips:

Start out slow until you get the form and rhythm correct. Next, speed up so that you are actually jumping from one foot to the other. Note that in the part where you bring your left leg to your right leg, before your left foot fully touches the floor, your right foot is already partially lifted. As your right leg goes back and lands (on the ball of foot), only then should the left foot fully rest on the floor. The grip on the handle is not as important as actually doing the exercise correctly and dynamically. If, however, you are a martial artist and have some specific punches in your regimen, then you adjust the hand and arm in such a way that it will very much resemble your way of punching. For example, in my style of karate, the arm opposite of the punching arm is pulled back so that the hand is above the chest and the palm is up.

Breathing technique:

Exhale as you row your arm and inhale as you release the pulley and switch grips.

Sports applications:

Any kind of sport that involves explosive leg work and hip joint flexibility will benefit from alternated dynamic lunges. We can mention running (especially the push-off phase in short-distance runs), racquet sports (reaching out for the ball in tennis), and gymnastics (improved flexibility and muscle strength for doing splits). The upper body rowing motion is particularly beneficial in rowing sports, also tennis and badminton (backhands). For martial artists, this fast, alternated row will prove essential in the rearing up (withdrawing of the arm after punch) motion and will benefit the whole punching movement in general (even more so when sport-specific modifications are applied to it).

Come on, warrior, you're not done yet!/progression:

IDP2:

Jump into the air while doing this so both of your feet are off the ground while switching grips. This will improve your dynamic balance and orientation even more.

> Master Crunch
>
> Difficulty level: A
>
> Caution: If you have back problems, you may be able to perform the exercise modification provided.
>
> Origin: ID
>
> Presenter: Self

Starting position:

Adjust the cable pulley to the lowest level or anchor an elastic band to a pulley station. Lie on a mat on your right buttock. Tightly grasp the cable handle or band handle with your left hand. The back of your right arm will be resting on the mat (note: in the picture you will see a dumbbell in my right hand because I was doing the progression described below).

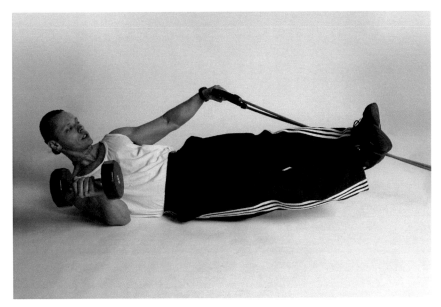

Photo 2.35

Next, turn your head toward your legs, tighten up the left side (oblique muscles), and lift up your legs. Hold your legs together and raise the upper body so that neither the right shoulder blade nor the lower back touch the mat (see Photo 2.35).

Movement:
Commence by raising your left arm holding the band and stretching the band (this will tighten your left side even more) upward until it is about perpendicular to the floor (see Photo 2.36). Try to lift your legs and upper body higher than the starting position. Then, lower your left arm, slightly reduce the tension in the left oblique muscles (sides), and lower your legs with the upper body (but still do not touch the mat!). Perform 15 repetitions and switch sides.

Major muscles involved:
In the arm that's rising, the medial deltoid is working (outer shoulder). The oblique muscle is working on the side that's crunching. In the arm that's holding the dumbbell, your biceps femoris is at work.

Ark's tips:
Make sure the Side Crunch position is correct. When your legs are bent and you lower your legs to the floor, you will not work the sides effectively. Also, make sure that the hand that's holding a dumbbell does not open much past 90 degrees.

Breathing technique:
Exhale when you raise the arm and inhale upon its return.

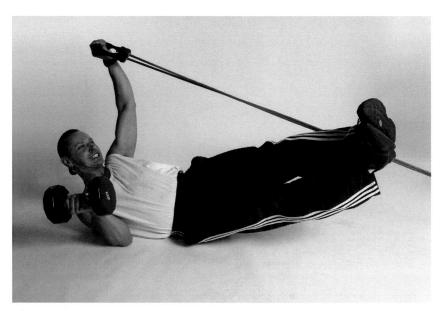

Photo 2.36

Sports applications:
The Master Crunch will prove effective for all athletes who throw overhead for maximum distance (javelin throwers, football quarterbacks, etc.), hit overhead (smash in tennis, or serving), or reach overhead (basketball, volleyball). For martial artists, we may mention that this exercise will help in punching (karate, boxing), kicking, and even wrestling moves. In karate or boxing, you rely on the oblique muscles to facilitate trunk rotation, and the Master Crunch will strengthen them. As far as the side arm raise part of the Master Crunch is concerned, it will be effective for basketball players (rebounding), volleyball players (e.g., in blocking), and in football tackles.

Come on, warrior, you're not done yet!/progression:

IDP1:
Instead of using your right arm as a support, hold a somewhat heavy dumbbell in it (as seen in the photos above). The arm should be bent at 90 degrees or more. Hold it tensed up for the duration of the set and then relax and switch hands. Note that the isometric contraction occurring here in the biceps will specifically help in throwing uppercuts in karate or any other martial arts that utilize uppercuts. Why? Because in karate, uppercuts do not utilize a full-range flexion or extension of the arm. This IDP will strengthen the biceps in the final stage of an uppercut.

Modification (for extension-biased persons[12]):
Lie on your side and perform a Side Crunch with only the shoulder blade coming off the mat (when you lie on the right side, the right shoulder blade will come off).

Crouching Tiger

Difficulty level: A

Caution: If you have knee problems, you may be able to perform the exercise modification provided.

Origin: K

Presenter: Warrior Susan

Starting position:

Squat down so that you stay on the balls of your feet and almost sit on your heels. Your hands will be used as support in the whole movement. Place them in front of you on the floor. You can actually stay on your fingers (see Photo 2.37).

Movement:

Partially straighten out your left leg (the other leg staying bent in the air and getting in the position for a back kick), look over your right shoulder, slightly turn your left foot clockwise, and deliver a right backside kick (see Photos 2.38–39). Return to the starting position. Now do the opposite. Partially straighten out the right leg, look over the left shoulder, slightly turn right foot counterclockwise, and deliver a left back kick. This counts as one repetition. Perform 15 repetitions on each side.

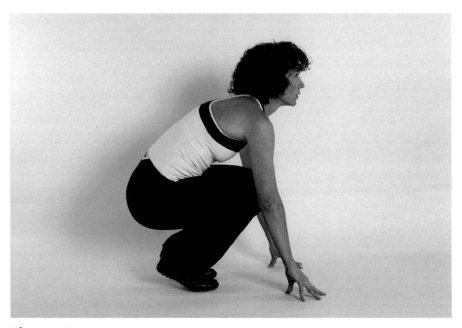

Photo 2.37

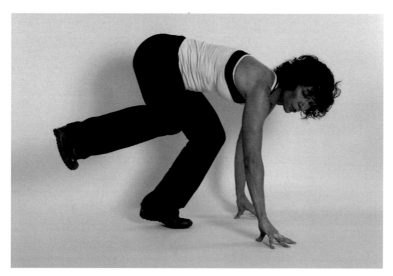

Photo 2.38

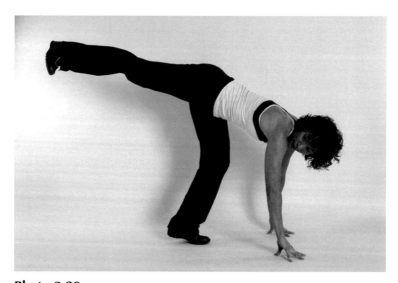

Photo 2.39

Major muscles involved:
In the lower body, the prime mover is your quadriceps (front thigh). In the midsection, the gluteus maximus (butt) and extensor spinae (lower back) stabilize the upper body so the leg can execute the kick.

Ark's tips:
Start exhaling when you're lifting yourself up on one leg. The final exhalation phase occurs when you deliver the kick. Inhale as you quickly return to a crouching position.

Breathing technique:
Exhale as you start straightening out the leg. The final portion of the exhalation should occur during the kick. Quickly breathe in as you go back to the initial position (crouching down with your hands down on the floor).

Sports applications:
This exercise will prove very useful, especially to the martial artists. Almost all kicks in the martial arts utilize either the front thigh or butt muscles. So, although this kick is not popular, it will strengthen the specific areas responsible for delivering devastating kicks.

Come on, warrior, you're not done yet!/progression:

IDP1:
Perform a double back kick but make the second one of a limited range of motion. What I mean is that after the first kick, return halfway back and execute the second kick. Then return the leg all the way down to the floor.

Modification (for persons with knee conditions):
Hold on to a stationary cable station, stand on one foot, and lift the knee of the other leg to the side and up. Try to bring the knee to your stomach. Make sure the leg is bent sufficiently and then extend it out in a kicking motion (kick with the outer edge of foot). Do not go fast. Try to squeeze muscles in the thigh and butt as you come to complete the kick. Hold for a split second and then return the knee to the initial position. Switch legs.

Okay, now, let's repeat this sequence twice more before we move on to sequence 3!

DESCRIPTIONS OF EXERCISES IN THE INTERMEDIATE PROGRAM, SEQUENCE 3

Flying Eagle/Isometric Lunge with Inverted Fly

Difficulty level: I

Caution: If you have back problems, you may be able to perform the exercise modification provided.

Origin: IDP

Presenter: Self

Starting position:
Stand in a left lead or right lead ready position holding two light dumbbells in a neutral grip (hands toward each other). See Photo 2.40.

Movement:
Begin by stepping forward with one foot and getting into a lunge position. In the lunge position, the front foot rests on the floor and is bent at 90 degrees, whereas the back foot rests on its ball and is bent at approximately 90 degrees as well (see Photo 2.41). Normally in a lunge, you would keep your upper body erect; however, here, you bend at the hips so that you are

almost parallel to the floor (face down). Next, lift your arms so that they are aligned with your bent-over torso (see Photos 2.42–43). Make sure you hold the dumbbells palms down. Perform 15 repetitions. In the next round when you get to this exercise in the circuit, remember to switch legs.

Major muscles involved:
In the upper body, you work the posterior deltoids (rear shoulders), trapezius (middle and upper), and rhomboids (middle back). In the lower body, you work all of the leg muscles.

Ark's tips:
Keep your back arched (not rounded) so that you work all of the back muscles. Do not bend your arms too much as this will compromise the effectiveness of the exercise. As you lift the arms, the angle between your upper body and the back of your arm/s should be around 90 degrees.

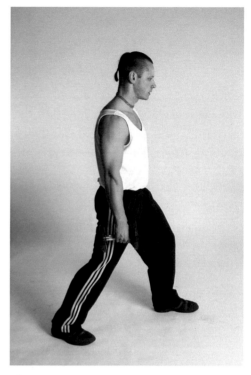

Photo 2.40

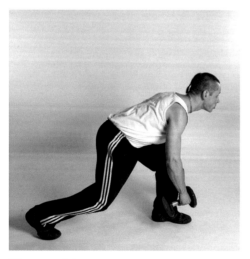

Photo 2.41

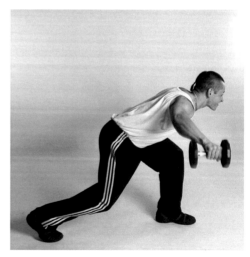

Photo 2.42

Breathing technique:
Exhale as you raise your arms and inhale as you lower them.

Sports applications:
The usefulness of this exercise will prove itself in rowing sports, gymnastics, tennis, racquetball, etc. The Flying Eagle will also strengthen your legs isometrically because you will stand in a lunge position for the duration of the entire set (15 reps). It will help in executing very basic sports skills, such as jumping for height or distance, any form of running or kicking (martial arts), and in pushing with the lower body (in swimming when changing direction and pushing away from the wall).

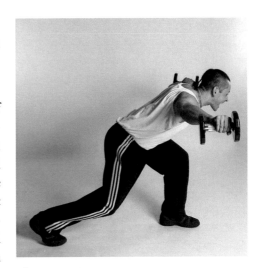

Photo 2.43

Come on, warrior, you're not done yet!/progression:

IDP2:
Perform the exercise standing on one foot only.

Modification (for extension-biased persons[13]):
Lie on a flat bench and perform inverted Flies.

> Parasurama's Power Punch/One armed Triceps Push-off
>
> Difficulty level: A
>
> Caution: If you have shoulder problems, you may be able to perform the exercise modification provided.
>
> Origin: ID
>
> Presenter: Warrior Marcin

Starting position:
Find an incline bench or a flat bench that you can slant. The bench should be adjusted so that it forms a 135-degree angle with the floor. Face the bench. Make sure it is positioned between your legs and place the opened palm of your left hand in front of you approximately chest high (as in a ready position to catch yourself from a fall). You may place the other hand on guard (as if you were protecting your jaw and ribs against a punch). See Photo 2.44.

Movement:

With the left palm extended out in front of you and the left elbow close to your side, begin falling down onto the bench. At that point, your heels will come off the floor and you will be standing on the balls of the feet. In the last moment, catch yourself from hitting the bench by tightening your whole arm and core and landing on the base of your palm (see Photos 2.45–46). Immediately push off, generating as much force as possible in the shortest amount of time (see Photo 2.47). Fall down onto the bench. Keep your shoulders aligned (parallel to the bench), while landing and pushing off. Do 15 push-offs on each side.

Major muscles involved:

As this exercise is very specific to punching sports (karate, kickboxing, etc.), you will need to keep the elbow close to your side (almost touching it). In this way, you will involve the very same muscles in

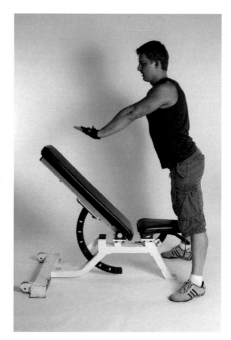

Photo 2.44

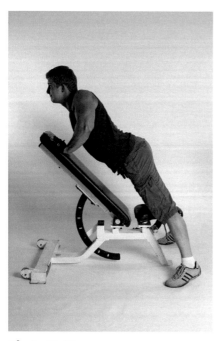

Photo 2.45

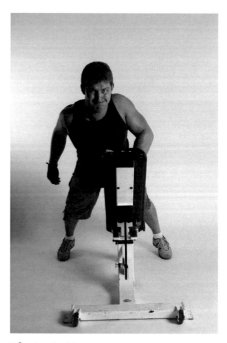

Photo 2.46

the same way as in a punch. Triceps brachii (back of arm) is the prime mover and clavicular pectoralis (upper chest) is the assisting mover in the exercise. Anterior deltoid (front shoulder) is assisting in the movement. Core muscles (abdominals, obliques), as well as sides of the back (latissimus dorsi), are stabilizing the trunk to make the pushing motion possible.

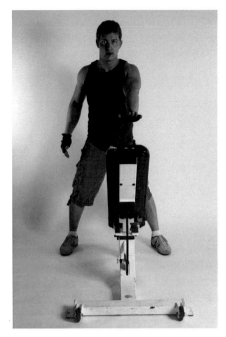

Photo 2.47

Ark's tips:

Focus on exploding, warrior! Don't spare your energy for what's to come. Generate as much strength as possible within that split second that you have and powerfully push yourself off. Visualize hitting an opponent or breaking a hard object or even the bench itself. But do not compromise proper form. Keep those shoulders aligned! Keep yourself very tight, rock-solid, including neck, especially when you come in contact with the bench.

Breathing technique:

Inhale as you drop your body on the bench and forcefully exhale as you push off the bench.

Sports applications:

Here is a perfect exercise for developing explosiveness of one's punch. More than anything, you will improve your starting strength[14] by doing Parasurama's Power Punch as well as the descend phase (eccentric strength[15]), and transition phase (amortization[16]). Other sport disciplines that will benefit from the triceps push-off are football (pushing), tennis (forehand), and gymnastics (free exercises).

Come on, warrior, you're not done yet!/progression:

IDP1:

Make a fist and try to land and push off from the first two knuckles. This will make the exercise more karate specific and strengthen the wrist for punches. Use a neutral fist position, that is, with the right palm of the hand facing to the left side.

Modification:
Use two arms when pushing off.

>   Eccentric Sit-up with Medicine Ball on Incline Bench

>   Difficulty level: A

>   Caution: If you have back problems, you may be able to perform the exercise modification provided.

>   Origin: IDP

>   Presenter: Warrior Kim G.

Starting position:
Sit on an incline bench with a medium weight medicine ball held in two hands. Hold the ball close to your chest (see Photo 2.48).

Movement:
Contract abdominal muscles and begin slowly lowering your upper body until shoulder blades almost touch the bench (see Photos 2.49–51). Next, rise up only until about 65 degrees from the bench, briefly pause, and slowly return to the down position. The sitting-up phase (concentric) should take you a second and the lowering phase (eccentric) should take you 5 seconds. Count to five and without pausing, sit up again. Repeat 10 times.

Major muscles involved:
You will work the upper portion[17] of the rectus abdominis (prime mover). Stabilizing muscles are the obliques.

Ark's tips:
You can almost hold[18] your breath while coming up. Then forcefully exhale and inhale and hold the breath again on your way down.

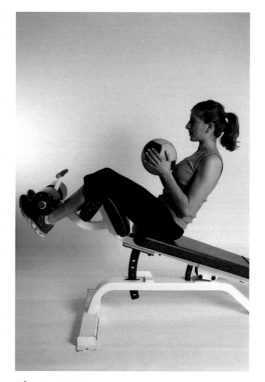

Photo 2.48

Breathing technique:
Slowly exhale as you come up, quickly inhale as you come to a stop, and again start breathing out slowly as you count down to five. Quickly inhale and begin coming up.

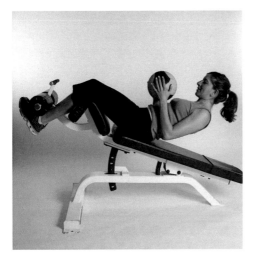

Photo 2.49

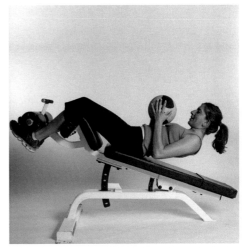

Photo 2.50

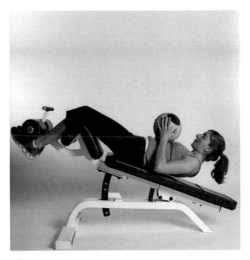

Photo 2.51

Sports applications:

Athletes whose main objective is throwing (baseball, javelin, etc.) will benefit from this exercise, as well as gymnasts.

Come on, warrior, you're not done yet!/progression:

IDP2:

Extend the eccentric portion to about 10 seconds and the concentric portion to about 2 seconds.

Modification (for extension-biased persons[19]):
While lying on a mat, perform a Crunch. Make sure that only your shoulder blades come off the mat and the small of your back remains flat.

Balarama's Squats

Difficulty level: I

Origin: ID

Presenter: Warrior Rich

Starting position:
Attach a medium tension elastic band to a pulley station. The pulley station should be set at medium height so that when you squat down (to about a sitting position or higher), the place where the band is attached aligns with your shoulders. Stand up straight to the side of the pulley and firmly grasp the elastic band with your left hand. Grab a light dumbbell with your right hand, lift up your right arm, and bend your elbow so that the dumbbell's left end is touching the sternum (chest area). See Photo 2.52. The right arm's position will not change for the duration of the set.

Movement:
Leaving the left hand grasping the band, step out to the right with your right foot and end up in a medium squat stance with feet parallel to one another (check feet position if necessary). As you are almost done squatting, your left hand will have extended so that the band will be stretched (see Photo 2.53). This tension

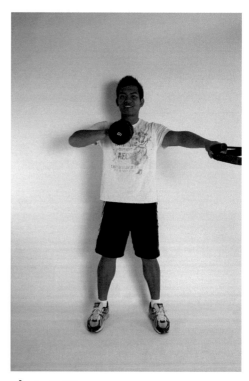

Photo 2.52

in the band will allow you to perform a Biceps Curl with your left arm. Perform this curl in an elbow-up, palm-down position (same as the right arm holding the dumbbell). See Photo 2.54. Repeat 15 times and switch sides.

Major muscles involved:
In the lower body, you are using the same muscles as in the squat exercise, such as front (quadriceps) and back of thigh (biceps femoris/hamstring). In the upper body, you work biceps brachii (front of arm).

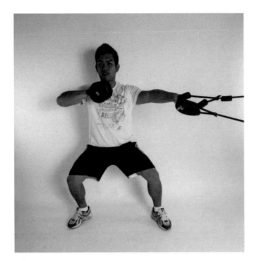 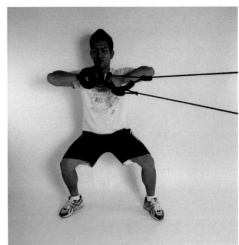

Photo 2.53   **Photo 2.54**

Ark's tips:
After you get in a squat position, maintain contracted muscles, especially in the core and arms, so that the curl will be performed properly.

Breathing technique:
Begin exhaling as you step out. Because the exercise is done in a fast manner, your exhalation will be complete after you curl with the arm. Inhale as you go back to a neutral stance.

Sports applications:
Any sport that requires muscle endurance in the shoulder area will benefit from the Balarama squats. Take boxing or karate, for example. In sparring matches or fighting, the *karateka* is required to keep hands up on guard at all times (in Kyokushin karate, it is so even when delivering a kick), which requires one to constantly maintain a state of isometric contraction in the muscles and execute powerful motions every few seconds. This calls for muscular endurance of certain muscle fibers.

Come on, warrior, you're not done yet!/progression:

IDP2:
Change position of the right arm to an "elbow in military press" position; that is, your elbow is in front of you instead of to the side. Your elbow is aligned with your right shoulder, and the angle between the right biceps and forearm is approximately 90 degrees. Hold this position as you are curling with the other arm.

Great, now, let's repeat this sequence twice more and then record our completion time.

Cooldown. Walk around for a minute and perform stretches for the muscles worked during the training session, such as back and front shoulders, biceps, triceps (back of arm), abdominals, etc.

Ending meditation:
This is the same as for the Beginner Krishna Warrior Challenge program.

Word of instruction:
Congratulations! You have just completed the second workout plan. Do you feel empowered now? Continue with it for the next 6 weeks, three times a week, each time trying to better your form and take less rest. Write down your completion times on your Personal Record Sheet (see Chapter 5). On other days, engage yourself in jogging, sports of your liking, or skill training that you may need for your specific discipline (football or soccer practice, performing kata or forms in karate). Continue eating in accordance with your body type 7 days a week. Make sure to take 1 day of complete rest.

FINAL ASSIGNMENTS

1. Perform a fitness assessment on yourself or have someone do it for you. See how much fat weight you've lost and how many pounds of lean muscle you've gained.

2. If you gained muscle and lost body fat, you will need to increase your protein intake to keep making gains (increase strength, power, etc.) and burning more fat. If you are a competitive athlete, you should try to apply protein recommendations that your body type requires (see Chapter 4) as well as necessary supplements (e.g., L-glutamine, etc.).

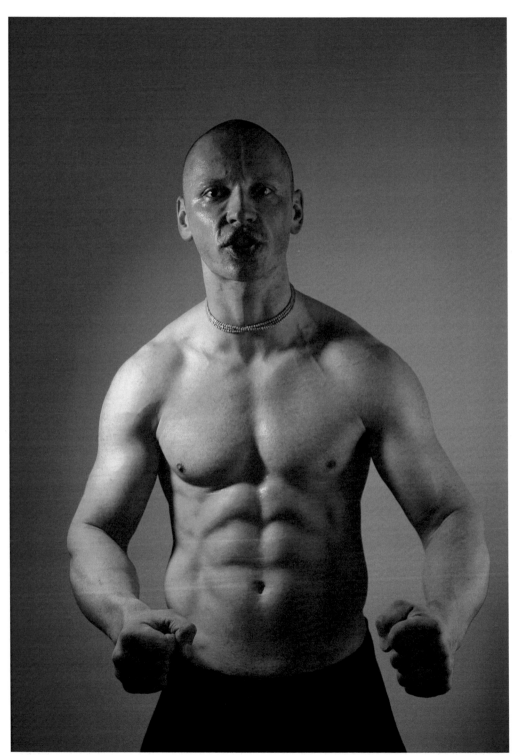

It is time to come to the next level!

Chapter III

Advanced Krishna Warrior Program

THE CASTLE OF MIND

"He who is regulated in his habits of eating, sleeping, recreation, and work can mitigate all material pains by practicing the yoga system [connecting in spirit with Krishna through one's work]."

Bhagavad-Gita 6.17

The lights in the training hall were dim. Goru sat down to meditate. I could only hear the deep inhalations and quick exhalations. After a while, the boy stood up and looked at me in anticipation, then at the half-man, half-lion Narasimhadeva, and then at me again.

"Are you ready for the workout of your life, Goru?"

There was silence for a moment, and then a car accelerating with great speed could be heard outside. Then silence again. I looked at Goru intently, and the boy looked at Lord Narasimhadeva.

"No, Ark. I can't pacify my mind. I just keep thinking about someone and what happened," Goru replied, rubbing his hands nervously.

"Do not worry, my friend. Did you harm anyone?"

"No, I disappointed someone. They got frustrated with me. They don't like me any—"

"That's all right . . ." I interjected. "You just stick to your warrior duty. You see, sometimes people, and your friends or even family, will expect you to compromise your schedule and/or principles, but generally, you should not. This will teach them a lesson that you are devoted to your training and principles. That will bring you respect in the long run."

"But—"

"There is no 'but', Goru, no 'but'! Only the PATH! Progress At The Highest," I yelled.

"And you will reach the Gift Of All Love (GOAL)!" he yelled back and looked down.

"Are you sure?" I gazed into his black eyes.

"Not so sure, Master Ark . . ." he sighed.

"How many times do I have to tell you not to address me . . ." I feigned anger.

"But you are . . ." Goru bit his lips and looked at Narasimhadeva.

"OK, dude, I did not sleep, and I ate a half of a large pepperoni pizza, double cheese . . . just 15 minutes ago. I feel out of it!"

"That's another thing. Because your recreation activity was off and you like that girl, everything else is off. Just don't talk to your mind anymore, OK? Don't let it replay that movie to you. That movie is over. OVER!" I rang the bell loudly by Goru's head to shock his mind.

Goru yelled like a crazy man: "I will become a fireeefighterrrr, the best I can ever be and no one will stray me away from the path I've chosen." He began the karate warm-up of running and push-ups.

Suddenly, the door opened and the receptionist appeared. "Mr. Madej, is everything all right?" She looked at me and kind of froze there, then stared at Goru for a moment. He already started a superset of Abhimanyu's pumps and One-armed Pull-ups.

I gave her a peaceful look and a nod and motioned with my hand to leave. She slowly exited.

SILVER DOOR 3: THE CASTLE OF INTELLIGENCE
REQUIRED ASSIGNMENTS

THE KRISHNA WARRIORS' CODE OF CONDUCT
A Krishna warrior knows by heart the code of conduct and can recite it when asked. He abides by it daily.

1. I shall refrain from unnecessary sensual enjoyment, which deviates me from the spiritual path:

   a) I will not indulge in eating meat or any other food not pleasing to the Lord and which has not first been offered to Him with love and devotion. I will offer Lord Krishna grains, vegetables, fruit, and milk products.

   b) I will not indulge in sex outside of marriage.

   c) I will not indulge in intoxication of any kind, including alcohol, drugs, coffee, or cigarettes.

   d) I will not gamble. All material necessities are met for those who worship the Lord with all their hearts.

2. I will rise early to chant the Lord's holy names, pray, and mediate so that He may give me strength to glorify Him with my life.

3. I will try to protect the physically and spiritually weak, both in word and action, as authorized by scripture and self-realized masters.

4. I will try to be polite and gentle among people, and I will not display physical or verbal aggression when there is no need for such.

5. I will be decisive and will not yield or conform to materialistic ways. Instead, I will practice the path of Krishna warriors and from that practice, derive strength to glorify the Supreme Warrior, God.

6. By all means, I shall avoid offending others who are fully engaged in the process of spiritual realization.

7. I will avoid unnecessarily criticizing or judging, knowing that I myself am not pure. If criticism becomes necessary, I will offer it personally, and not in public as if to demean.

BRONZE DOOR 3

ASSIGNMENTS:

1. *(Required)* If you have not already done so, adjust your food intake according to your body composition change.

2. *(Required)* Maintain your eating habits as in the 2nd phase.

3. *(Required)* Fill out your PAG for the third month (see Chapter 5). Continue with the Transcendental Warrior Achievement Program as described in the first chapter.

4. *(Optional)* If needed, modify your daily schedule with, most importantly, workout times and workout types included.

5. *(Optional)* Continue filling out your PRS (see Chapter 5).

GOLDEN DOOR 3

Meditation. Same as for the Beginner Krishna Warrior Fitness Challenge.

Warm-up. Duration of 5 minutes.

Presenters: Warriors Susan and Ark

Equipment needed: None

Execution:

Push-up, creep through (see Photos 3X.1–18), crab walk forward (2–3 steps), crab walk backward (2–3 steps), dip (not shown), turnover, come to a crouching position and explode up. Land in a crouching position and return to the push-up position. Repeat the whole sequence at least 15 times.

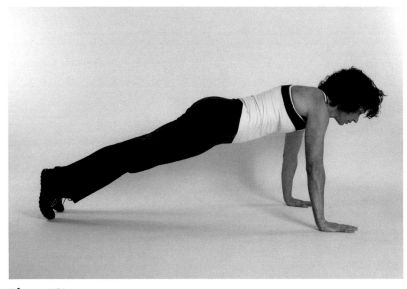

Photo 3X.1

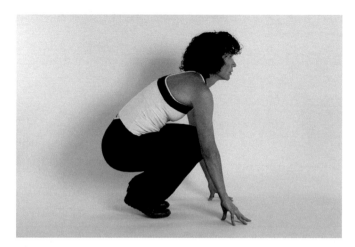

Photo 3X.2

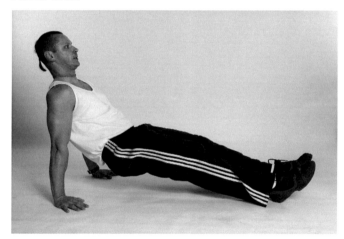

Photo 3X.3

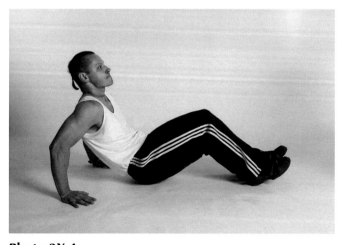

Photo 3X.4

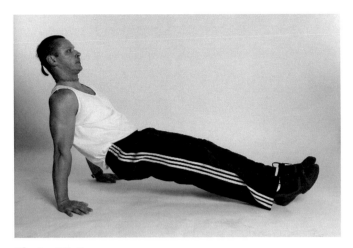

Photo 3X.5

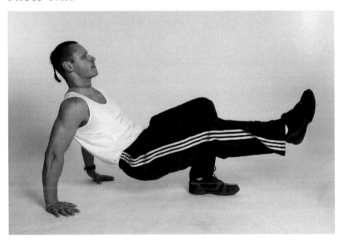

Photo 3X.6

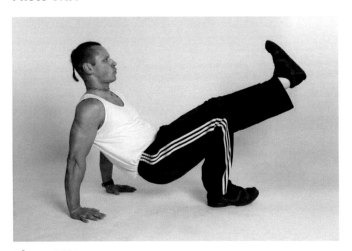

Photo 3X.7

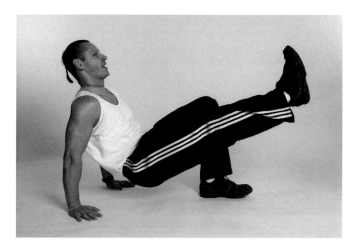

Photo 3X.8

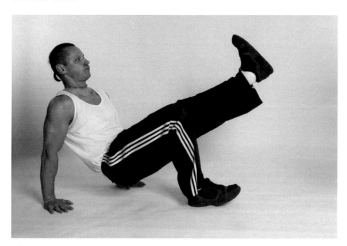

Photo 3X.9

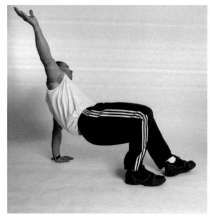

Photo 3X.10

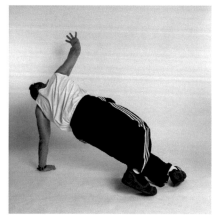

Photo 3X.11

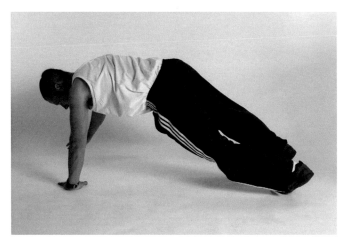

Photo 3X.12

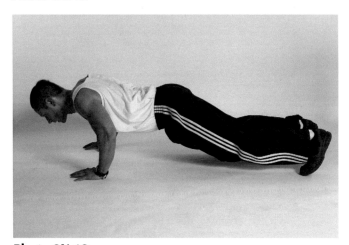

Photo 3X.13

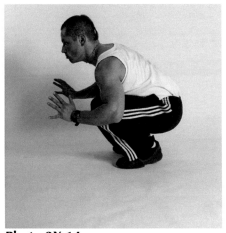

Photo 3X.14

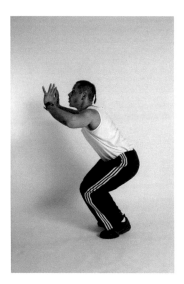

Photo 3X.15

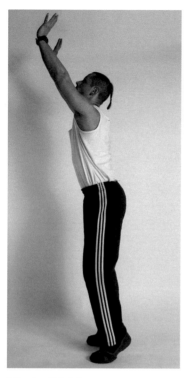

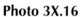

Photo 3X.17

Photo 3X.16

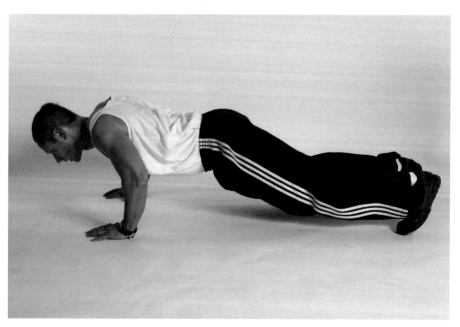

Photo 3X.18

Comments: By "creeping through," we mean literally walking on the balls of your feet (because you start in a push-up position), and then your heels, without taking your hands off the floor so you end up in the position seen in Photo 3X.2. When doing a dip, keep hips up. When doing the turnover, switch arms each time you do it.

Progression: Add more push-ups and more steps to your crab walk and explode twice instead of once.

EXERCISES IN THE MAIN CORE OF THE WORKOUT

Equipment needed: adjustable pulley station, stepper (with at least one riser), mat, elastic bands (one thick, one medium or light), a Smith's Machine, or a stable very low bar (to do a pull-up from supine position), stopwatch.

Estimated Completion Time: 55 minutes

General Comments: ECT listed above was calculated during a rather medium-paced workout. Time to quickly adjust pulleys and bands is included. Meditation and warm-up times are not included. If you go over 55 minutes, then you probably rested too long between exercises and/or sequences. Remember, the idea behind the PHA system of training is to go NONSTOP. For a competitive finishing time of the intermediate workout with my own loading parameters, see Chapter 5, Physical Assessments.

SEQUENCE 1 (REPEATED THREE TIMES IN CIRCUITLIKE FASHION):
    Reverse Tiger Push-ups
    Core Master
    Kunti's Kick
    Small Kangaroo Jumps

SEQUENCE 2 (REPEATED THREE TIMES IN CIRCUITLIKE FASHION):
    Explosive Push-ups on Steppers
    Hamstring Push-ups
    Cakra Wheel
    Karate Cracker Squats

SEQUENCE 3 (REPEATED THREE TIMES IN CIRCUITLIKE FASHION):
    Crocodile Walk
    Arjuna Tiger Pull
    Bhima Pull
    One-legged Squat

DESCRIPTIONS OF EXERCISES IN THE ADVANCED PROGRAM, SEQUENCE 1

Reverse Tiger Push-ups

Difficulty level: S

Origin: K

Presenter: Warrior Greg

Starting position:

Begin by getting into a regular push-up position, that is, supporting yourself on the palms of your hands and two feet. Feet can be spread at shoulder width; arms, fingers pointing forward and placed on the mat approximately shoulder width apart or a little wider (see Photo 3.1).

Movement:

Quickly inhale, shift your body forward so that the shoulders are positioned an inch or two further from your hands (see Photo 3.2). Lower the torso so that your chest is very close to the floor (see Photos 3.3–3.4). Hold your breath. Your elbows should be touching your sides (very narrow push-up position), and your hips should be higher than the rest of the upper body. Start exhaling, push back with your hands (your hips will come up even more), and using your abdominal muscles, shift the whole body back on your forearms until your head is aligned with your elbows (see Photos 3.5–3.6). Then, begin lifting up the arms, starting with your elbows, until you end up in the starting position (see Photos 3.7–3.8). Repeat the whole cycle 15 times.

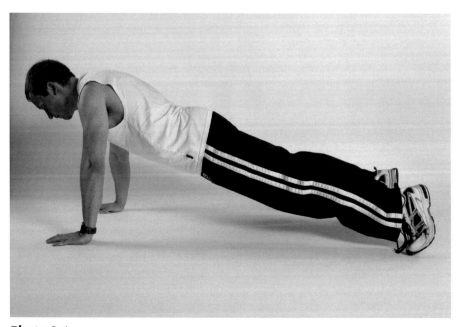

Photo 3.1

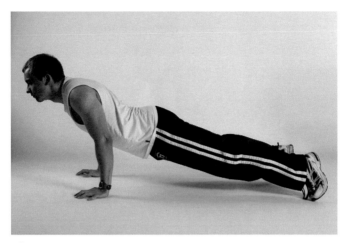

Photo 3.2

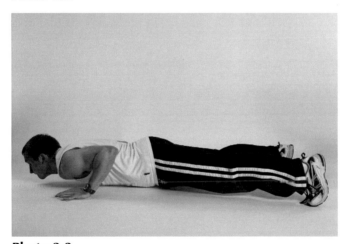

Photo 3.3

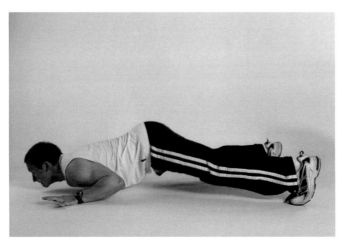

Photo 3.4

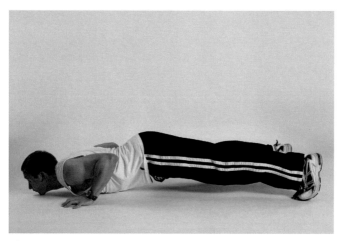

Photo 3.5

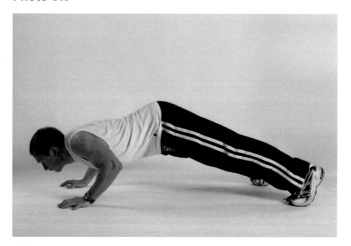

Photo 3.6

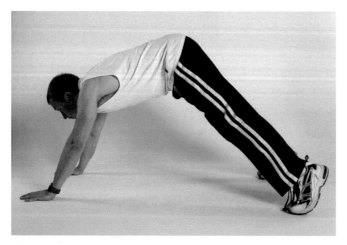

Photo 3.7

Major muscles involved:
There are many muscles at work here. Clavicular pectoralis muscles (upper chest) are involved, although you may not really feel them a lot. Triceps brachii (back of arm) is doing a tremendous amount of work at the pushing-up motion, and it is the prime mover in this exercise. Anterior deltoid (front shoulder) muscle is assisting the pectoralis and triceps brachii muscles in the pushing motion. The push-

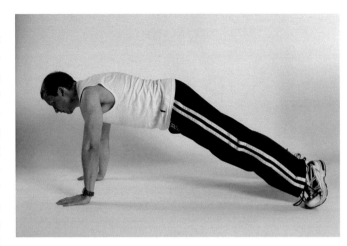

Photo 3.8

ing-up motion forces the rectus abdominis to stabilize your core, and thus a great amount of force is generated through that muscle. Another stabilizing muscle in Tiger Push-ups is latissimus dorsi (sides of back). Serratus anterior is also part of the stabilizing muscle group in Tiger Push-ups.

Ark's tips:
Just like in the Tiger Push-up, you should do the exercise quickly (although by its nature it will never be as fast as the former). After you get comfortable with the form and become stronger, you may slow down. Actually, this exercise will best serve its purpose (explosiveness) when done fast. Push from the bottom outer ends of your palms.

Breathing technique:
Inhale at the start of the exercise when you shift your body forward. Hold your breath as you get ready to push back from your wrists and forearms. After you get through the hardest part of the pushing back, you can start a forceful exhalation.

Sports applications:
Reverse Tiger Push-ups will benefit anybody whose sport discipline involves pushing, such as boxing (jab), martial arts (various punches)[20], football (linemen pushing, hitting, repelling), discus throwing, etc.

Come on, warrior, you're not done yet!/progression:

IDP1:

Rest on your knees and place one hand behind your back. Try to perform the same movement.

> Core Master
>
> Difficulty level: A
>
> Caution: If you have back problems, you may be able to perform the exercise modification provided.
>
> Origin: ID
>
> Presenter: Warrior Kim G.

Starting position:

Adjust the pulley to a position between high and medium (for shorter persons, the pulley should be lower than for tall persons). Adjust the weight so that it is somewhat light. Place a mat by the pulley, grab the handle of the pulley with your left hand, and sit on the mat facing the pulley (see Photo 3.9). Next, supporting yourself with your right hand placed on mat (but not forearm), raise both legs and hold them up straight in the direction of the pulley (see Photo 3.10). Put the chest up, tighten muscles in the mid- and lower back, then press down hard with your right hand so that your position is stable. Your body should resemble a standing letter "V" when seen from the side.

Movement:

Using a neutral grip (palm of the left hand will be turned right), perform a rowing motion, pulling the handle toward you. Then return your arm to its initial position (see Photos 3.11–12). This makes one repetition. Perform 15 of them on each arm.

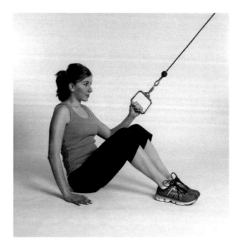

Photo 3.9

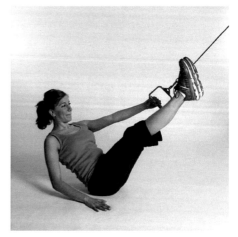

Photo 3.10

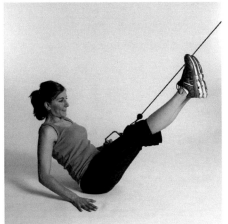

Photo 3.11   **Photo 3.12**

Major muscles involved:
Quite a few of them are involved here! First of all, the rowing motion works the latissimus dorsi (sides of back) and biceps brachii. By holding the "V" position, you work rectus femoris (upper front thigh), rectus abdominis (especially lower abdominals), and erector spinae (mid- and lower back).

Ark's tips:
Perform the movement at a medium tempo. In this exercise, it is all about control and keeping the muscles under great tension. Core Master is definitely not for power development or speed like many others in this book.

Breathing technique:
Exhale as you pull the handle toward you and inhale when you extend the arm back.

Sports applications:
The Core Master will be useful for all those who work on strengthening their trunk muscles. Sport disciplines like gymnastics, acrobatics, or even certain dances will benefit from Core Master exercise as it trains you to contract muscles isometrically (without flexing or extending) in a suspended position.

Come on, warrior, you're not done yet!/progression:

IDP1:
Take your right hand off the mat and hold a light dumbbell instead (use neutral grip). Hold it out to your side. Perform the same movement with the other arm.

Modification (for extension-biased persons[21]):
Place your right foot on the floor (knee bent at 90 degrees). Pull the cable with your right hand in the manner described above. You may need to decrease the angle between torso and legs by bending forward a little.

   Kunti's Kick/Side Kick with Band

   Difficulty level: A

   Origin: ID

   Presenter: Warrior Susan

Starting position:
Hold an elastic cord, band, or tube (versa cuff can also be used). Fold it once or twice (to create sufficient resistance) and loop it around your left foot. Holding with both hands the two ends of the cord, lift up your left leg so that it is bent at 90 degrees (see Photo 3.13). Find your point of balance.

Movement:
Holding the cord tightly with both hands and looking straight ahead, push through your hip and straighten your left leg to the side so that it is fully extended with toes pointing in front of you and heel pointing to the back (see Photos 3.14–15). Flex the leg back. Perform 15 Side Kicks in this manner.

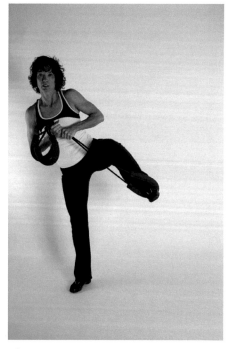

Photo 3.13

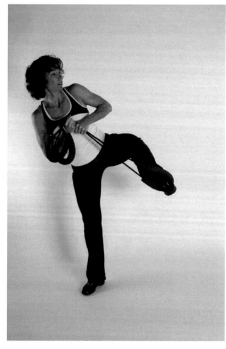

Photo 3.14

Major muscles involved:
In the lower body are the gluteus maximus (butt) and quadriceps (front of thigh). Gluteus maximus is assisting the thigh muscles in performing this side leg extension. Thigh muscles are the prime movers in the Side Kick. Core muscles (external obliques and rectus abdominis) are also involved in stabilizing the trunk in this unnatural position so that you can Side Kick without losing your balance. Also, gluteus maximus of the supporting leg is greatly involved to stabilize the whole weight of your body.

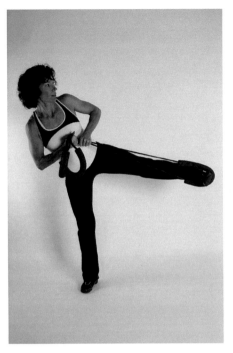

Ark's tips:
Make sure that throughout the movement (extending leg and taking it back), you maintain the line of your body with the center line, which is a line perpendicular to the floor. In other words, keep yourself erect and do not let your trunk deviate to the side (as is the tendency) to facilitate easier movement.

Photo 3.15

Breathing technique:
Exhale as you extend your leg and begin inhaling as you flex it back.

Sports applications:
This exercise will prove of great value to any combative artist or athlete who practices kicking to the side.

Come on, warrior, you're not done yet!/progression:

IDP1:
Instead of looking straight ahead, look at your extending leg. You will find that it is harder to stay in balance, but it will also be more specific to karate, or martial arts that utilize Side Kicks.

Small Kangaroo Jumps

Difficulty level: I

Caution: if you have knee problems, you may be able to perform the exercise modification provided.

Origin: K

Presenter: Warrior Kim D.

Starting position:
Assume a crouching position (squat down until you almost sit on your heels) with your hands in front. You are maintaining balance on the balls of your feet (see Photo 3.16).

Movement:
Suddenly jump up and forward, making sure to land on the balls of your feet (see Photos 3.17–20). Perform 20 jumps.

Major muscles involved:
The soleus and gastrocnemius of the back of the shin are involved as prime mover and assisting mover. Other muscles that aid in the jumping motion are vastus lateralis and vastus medialis (upper front thigh).

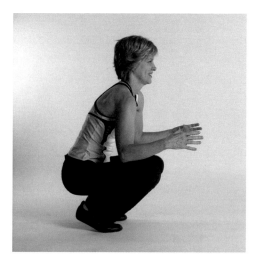

Photo 3.16

Breathing technique:
Rapidly exhale as you push off the floor and inhale as you are about to land.

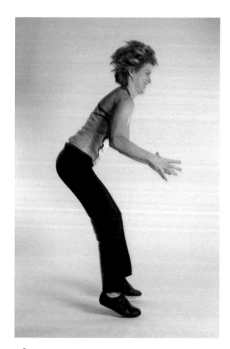

Photo 3.17

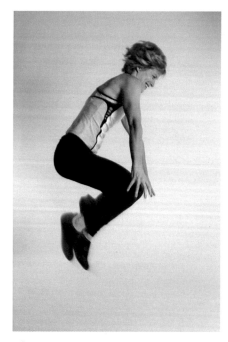

Photo 3.18

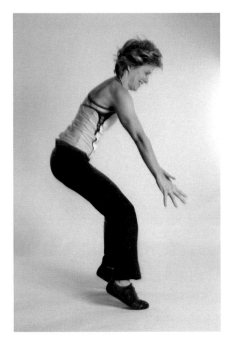

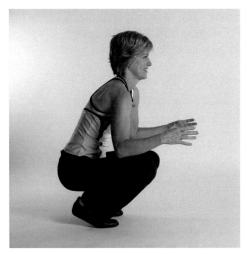

Photo 3.20

Photo 3.19

Sports applications:

The Small Kangaroo Jump will help all those who practice endurance-type or long-distance activities (walking, running, jumping). Because soleus muscle has more slow twitch fibers[22] than any other fiber, it will, therefore, be mainly used by those athletes. A well developed calf muscle will give you the final push in launching the body forward and up as seen in running, the high jump, long jump, etc.

Come on, warrior, you're not done yet!/progression:

IDP1:

Jump backwards or/and sideways (to the right and then left, 15 times each side).

Modification (for persons with knee problems):

Perform a simple partial squat; that is, bend your knees so that the angle between the back of your thigh and calf is approximately 135 degrees.

Okay, now let's repeat this sequence twice more before moving on to sequence 2!

DESCRIPTIONS OF EXERCISES IN THE ADVANCED PROGRAM, SEQUENCE 2

Explosive Push-ups on Steppers

Difficulty level: A

Caution: If you have shoulder or wrist problems, you may be able to perform the exercise modification provided.

Origin: IDP

Presenter: Warrior Greg

Starting position:
Place two steppers on the floor with at least two risers for each one. They should be placed slightly wider than your shoulder width. Get between the steppers in a standard push-up position (arms straight) but with each hand on top of stepper (fingers of each hand should face the same direction). Tighten up core muscles, wrists, and fingers (see Photo 3.21).

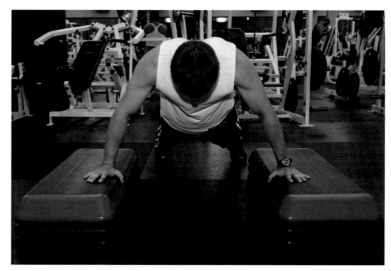

Photo 3.21

Movement:
Suddenly jump off the two steppers, bend arms, cushion the fall, and end up in a push-up position (arms bent) on the floor (mat) between steppers. While doing so, lift up one foot so you end up with only one leg supporting your lower body (see Photo 3.22). Even before you come to a complete stop, you must immediately propel yourself up with great force and end up in the starting position with your hands on two steppers and both feet down (see Photo 3.23). This counts as one explosive push-up. Repeat, this time alternating the foot being lifted (see Photos 3.24–25). Perform 15 push-ups.

Major muscles involved:
As in any push-up, the muscles involved would be the pectoralis group (chest), front shoulder (anterior deltoid), triceps brachii (back of arm), and core muscles (rectus abdominis, external oblique). Depending on whether you perform narrow or wide explosive push-ups,

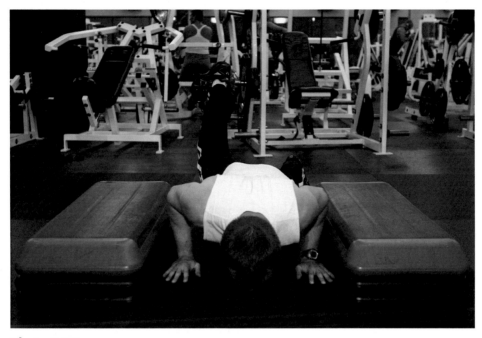

Photo 3.22

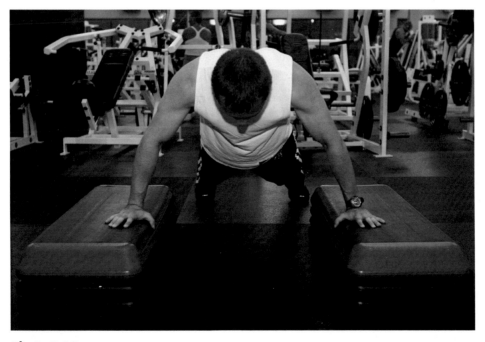

Photo 3.23

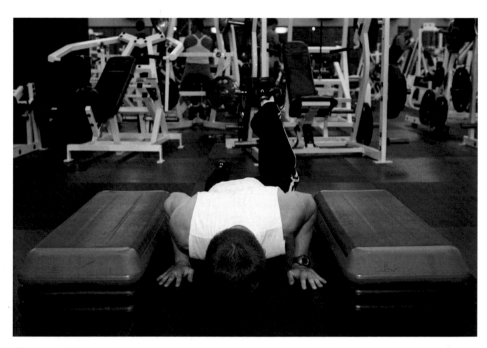

Photo 3.24

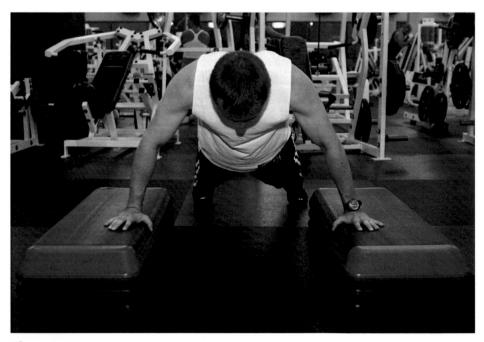

Photo 3.25

you will use certain muscles more than others (see alternated push-ups in the Beginner's Krishna Warrior program).

Ark's tips:
Here the key is to keep every single muscle very contracted, especially in the arms and core. Think "explode" before you even land between steppers. Synchronize breathing with movement. Make sure you cushion the fall by bending your arms before the hands come in contact with floor. At the same time, do not relax them excessively when you bend, unless you want to fall on your face. This exercise puts a lot of work on those fast twitch fiber muscles and requires a very good dynamic coordination between different muscles.

Breathing technique:
There will be a rapid exhalation as you jump off the steppers, and as your upper body is in the air, you quickly inhale. When your hands begin to land on the floor and you are in the so-called descend phase, you hold your breath momentarily and tighten up your arms and core area. As you begin to propel yourself back up and tension in the muscles has increased, start a powerful exhalation. Just before you find yourself on the two steppers again, rapidly inhale and stabilize your position. Exhale while jumping off again.

Sports applications:
Any kind of sport that involves explosive upper body movements will benefit from these push-ups. We may mention karate, other martial arts, wrestling, boxing, etc. Other kinds of sport disciplines that could use this exercise are tennis (forehand), gymnastics (free exercises), and football (pushing).

Come on, warrior, you're not done yet!/progression:

P2:
Add one more riser and work your way up to four or five.

Modification (for persons with shoulder and wrist conditions):
Perform regular push-ups on the floor without bending your arms more than 90 degrees.

> Hamstring Push-ups
>
> Difficulty level: I
>
> Origin: ID
>
> Presenter: Warrior Rich

Starting position:
Adjust a pulley station to a low setting and attach a power band to it (or an elastic band). Wrap the band around your left leg and get in a standard push-up position as shown in the photo (3.26). Make sure there is tension in the band when the leg is bent at a 90-degree angle. If there is no sufficient tension, you must move forward away from the cable station to stretch the band.

Movement:
Perform a regular push-up while tensing up left hamstring muscles and maintaining a right angle. See Photos 3.27–28. Do 15 push-ups. Remember to switch legs in the next round of the sequence.

Major muscles involved:
As in any push-up, the muscles involved would be the pectoralis group (chest) as prime movers, front shoulder (anterior deltoid), and triceps brachii (back of arm) as assisting movers, and core muscles (rectus abdominis, external oblique) as stabilizers. In addition, you are significantly working the biceps femoris (hamstring group/back of thigh) and gluteus maximus (buttock) muscles of the leg attached to the band.

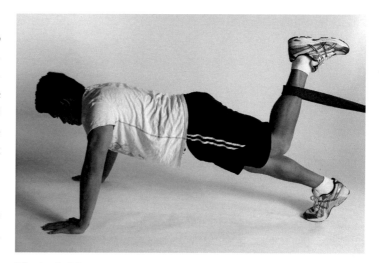

Photo 3.26

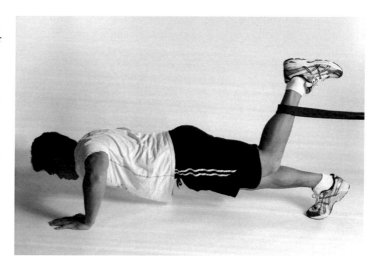

Photo 3.27

Ark's tips:
Keep your abdominals tight and slightly pushed in. Ensure that you are not hyperextending your back. Each time you come down to the floor, try to consciously contract the muscle in the back of left thigh (hamstring).

Breathing technique:
Exhale when pushing up and inhale on your way back.

Sports applications:
In addition to working arms and core, the Hamstring Push-up places emphasis on the lower back, glute (buttocks), and hamstring (back of thigh) muscles. By holding the

tension in the hamstring, you create a slightly arched position and that is why it will also help in all sports that require raising up with an arched back, such as weight lifting (rising out of the squat, dead lift), baseball (catching overhead balls), basketball (jumping for rebounds), volleyball (blocking or spiking), high jump, etc.

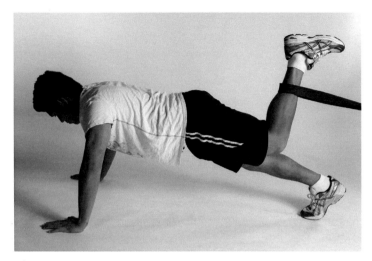

Photo 3.28

Come on, warrior, you're not done yet!/progression:

IDP1:

Have someone place a plate on your midback. Perform the same movement.

Cakra Wheel/Leg Circles Hanging Down from a Bar

Difficulty level: S

Caution: If you have back problems, you may be able to perform the exercise modification provided.

Origin: IDP

Presenter: Self

Starting position:

Using a medium to wide grip, hang down with your legs straight from a chin-up bar. You might want to use a stepper, wooden block, or a few weight plates to accommodate your height (see Photo 3.29). Basically, you will need to minimize dynamic movements in this exercise. Touching the floor after every repetition will help.

Movement:

Contract your abdominal muscles as hard as you can and lift your legs up and to the side. Execute a circle and slowly bring your legs down (see Photos 3.30–35). Touch the floor, or

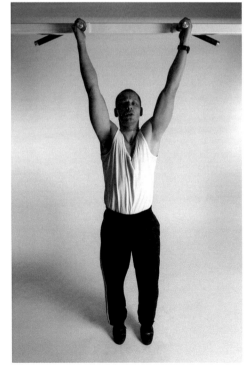

Photo 3.29

stepper, with your feet to lose dynamic momentum and start over. Perform eight circles each way (clockwise and counterclockwise).

Major muscles involved:
There is a lot of work for your hand and forearm muscles (e.g., flexor carpi, flexor pollicis brevis, extensor carpi, etc.) because you rely on them to hold you up. And there are a number of muscles in the forearm, some of which manipulate your fingers and elbows. The main muscle performing the movement, however, is rectus abdominis (abdominals), and the assisting muscles in the core are external obliques (sides), iliopsoas, and the pectineus (hip flexors).

Ark's tips:
The fuller the circle, the better. To get the most out of this exercise, perform it at a medium to slow tempo.

Breathing technique:
Hold your breath just so you get the legs up in the air. Next, start exhaling as you make the whole circle. Inhale and repeat.

Sports applications:
Sports that require athletes to raise their legs high in front of body will benefit from the Cakra Wheel. We may mention here karate, gymnastics, modern dance, soccer, football, etc.

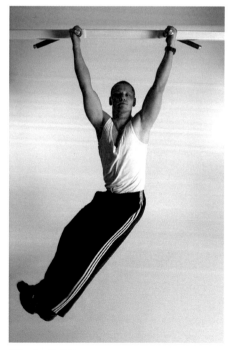

Photo 3.30

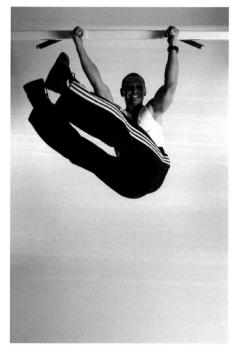

Photo 3.31

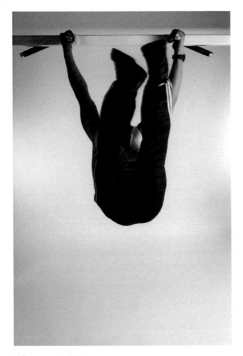

Photo 3.32

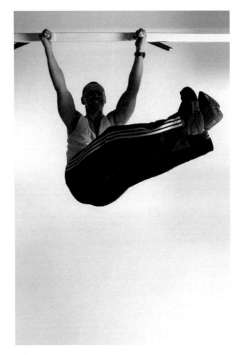

Photo 3.33

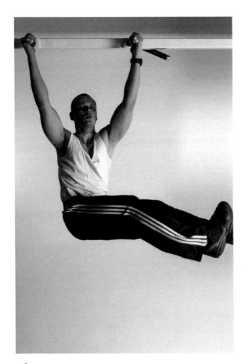

Photo 3.34

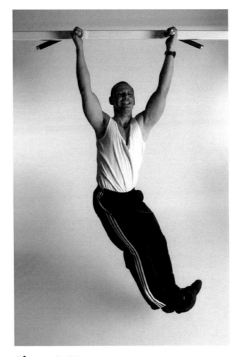

Photo 3.35

Come on, warrior, you're not done yet!/progression:

IDP2:
Slow down the movement even more and/or try to hold it at nine and three o'clock.

Modification (for extension-biased persons[23]):
Perform a simple Crunch. Make sure only the shoulder blades come off the mat while the small of the back stays flat.

> Karate Cracker Squats
>
> Difficulty level: I
>
> Caution: If you have knee problems, you may be able to perform the exercise modification provided.
>
> Origin: K
>
> Presenter: Warrior Kim D.

Starting position:
Squat down on your left leg to the side so that you are literally sitting on your heel (see Photos 3.36–37). The foot of the leg you are squatting on is flat. The right leg is straight and its toes are pointing to the ceiling. Your trunk, including the head, is shifted forward

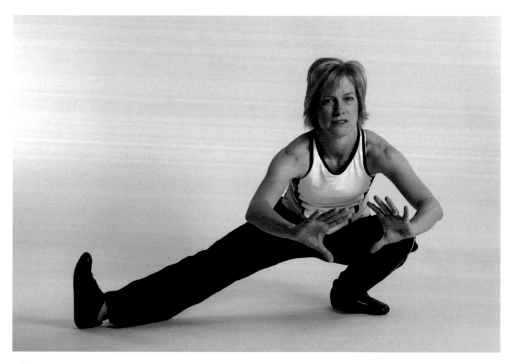

Photo 3.36

a little bit in relation to the rest of the body. Place your arms in front of you to establish balance (the tendency for your body is to tip backward just because you are sitting very low on your heel).

Movement:
Commence by squeezing left obliques (sides of trunk), rectus abdominis (abdominals), and muscles of the left leg, including your left gluteus maximus (buttock), in order to stand back up (see Photo 3.38). Immediately switch position to your right leg. Push yourself back up and squat down on your left again. Each time you perform two such squats (left and right squat), they count as one repetition. Perform 15 repetitions in this manner.

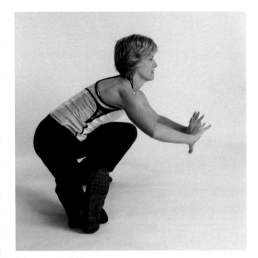

Photo 3.37

Major muscles involved:
Here is a great exercise for the outer thighs! In the squatting leg, you work the quadriceps (front of thigh or four major muscles located there) and hamstrings (back of thigh, specifically biceps femoris). These are your prime movers and assisting movers. In the trunk section, you work your oblique muscles (on the squatting leg side), as well as abdominals (rectus abdominis). They are stabilizing the trunk for you. Gluteus medius and gluteus maximus (buttocks) are also involved in the assisting job (the squatting leg side).

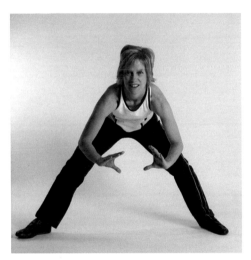

Photo 3.38

Ark's tips:
The most important thing in this exercise is to begin and complete each squat on a flat foot (the other foot is, of course, pointing up to the ceiling). Maintain an even and moderate tempo. When you come up, do not straighten legs up all the way. You can maintain a partial squat (see Photo 3.38) during switching, and in this way, maintain constant tension in the muscles worked.

Breathing technique:
Exhale as you start coming up on one leg and inhale as you land on the opposite leg.

Sports applications:
Karate Cracker Squats will help an athlete in the execution of foundational skills such as jumping for height or distance, running, various kicks, or pushing with the lower body. We can mention sports like basketball (shooting), the high jump, volleyball (jumping to spike), bounding, football, soccer, and many kicks in the martial arts.

Come on, warrior, you're not done yet!/progression:

IDP1:
Hold a plate in front of you and perform the movement.

Modification (for persons with knee conditions):
Perform the same exercise but with a limited range of motion in the knee, or perform partial squats as described in the Karna's Fall exercise modification.

Great, now let's repeat this two more times before going to the final sequence!

DESCRIPTIONS OF EXERCISES IN THE ADVANCED PROGRAM, SEQUENCE 3

Crocodile Walk

Difficulty level: A

Caution: If you have shoulder problems, you may be able to perform the exercise modification provided.

Origin: K

Presenter: Warrior Marcin

Starting position:
Find a spacious area somewhere away from the machines. If the gym is not crowded and people are not passing by you all the time, you could use an aisle between the rows of machines. Get in a push-up position on your knees (see Photo 3.39). Next, bend your left knee and move it up and to the side. Move the right hand slightly forward and the left hand slightly back (see Photos 3.40–41). It helps if both hands are turned in slightly. Lower your upper body as if you were going to perform a push-up. At this point, the inner side of the left knee and back of the left triceps (slightly above the elbow) should almost touch. If they are too far apart, you should then lower your upper body more. Extend out your right leg so that it is perfectly straight and it is resting on the toes. Now, contract the muscles in the core and arms while bringing the upper body even closer to the floor so that your chin almost brushes the floor (keep your head up so that you see the floor directly ahead of you). The foot of the left leg is resting on the large toe and partially on the side of the ball of the foot. The knee is turned out. The back of your arm (triceps brachii) and inside of the knee could press against one another. Your right arm is in front in relation to the left arm, and it is even more directed to the outside. You will feel the tension in the arms and right side of the torso increase. Hold your breath momentarily.

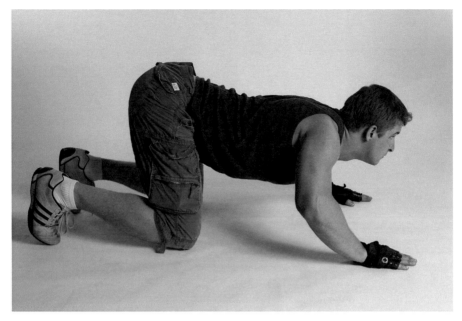

Photo 3.39

Movement:

Push off from your left leg and right arm and simultaneously start to bend your right leg, bringing it forward, moving your right arm forward and straightening out the left leg (see Photos 3.42–45). Your right arm will stay in the same place. The idea is to end up in exactly the opposite position; that is, with the right leg bent and touching the back of the right arm, your left leg straight and your left arm is forward. That counts as one repetition. Do 15 Crocodiles.

Major muscles involved:

How about all of them? Warriors, the Crocodile Walk is one of the most total exercises you have ever tried and ever will try! It is hard to think of a more total body exercise. It focuses on the upper body and midsection. First of all, the exercise creates a tremendous amount of muscle tension in the triceps brachii (back of the arm). This muscle is the prime mover for the

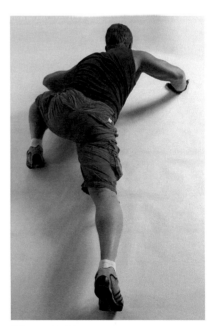

Photo 3.40

upper body. The stabilizers for the upper body are your chest (pectorals), anterior deltoids (front of shoulder), and latissimus dorsi (sides of back). The muscles that stabilize your trunk during this movement are: rectus abdominis (abdominals), obliques (one of them at a time,

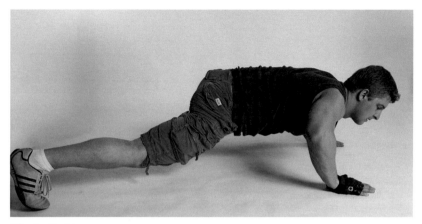

Photo 3.41

because the other oblique muscle is assisting the leg in moving forward, so it is an assisting mover), teres major (upper back), trapezius (upper back), latissimus dorsi (midback), and erector spinae (lower back). Some of the muscles just mentioned also perform the function of assisting movers (for example, teres major and middle trapezius, when moving the arm up and forward). Posterior deltoid (rear shoulder) also performs two functions here; it helps to move the arm when it is traveling forward, and it powerfully stabilizes the arm when it is time to land. In the lower body, the prime work is performed by the front thigh muscles such as vastus medialis, lateralis, etc.

Ark's tips:
It is better to do this exercise correctly or not do it at all. That is why I included it in the most advanced phase of Krishna warrior training. You require a very strong upper body, and your wrists have to be very adapted to this amount of stress. Therefore, don't jump to this phase before you have mastered the beginner and intermediate levels. Keep your whole body very low, just above the floor. Visualize that you are actually crawling and you do not have any room above your head. Better yet, visualize an electric wire that is just an inch or two above your head. If you go too high, you get shocked! Keep your muscles strongly contracted throughout the movement. Some muscles in your body will work less at some points, but most of the whole musculature is under constant tension. That's why it's a great exercise! Taste it!

Breathing technique:
Hold your breath when you begin pushing off with your left leg and right arm. Once you get the movement going, start to quickly exhale. When you land in the opposite position, rapidly breathe in. Hold your breath again, maximally contract your muscles in the arms and stomach, and push off again.

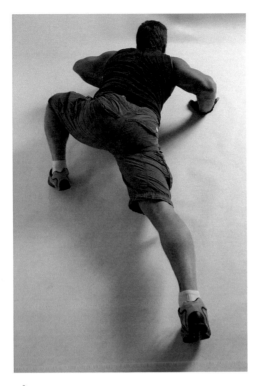

Photo 3.42

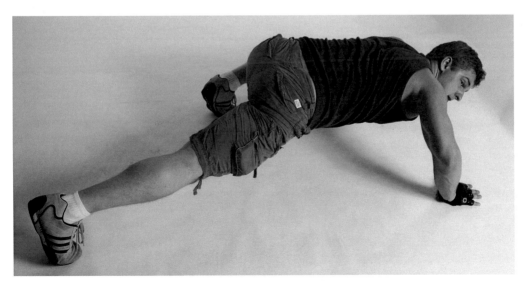

Photo 3.43

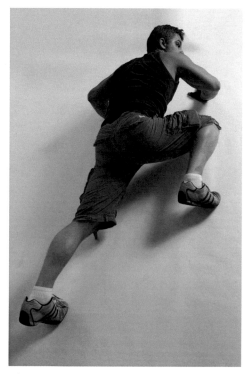

Photo 3.44

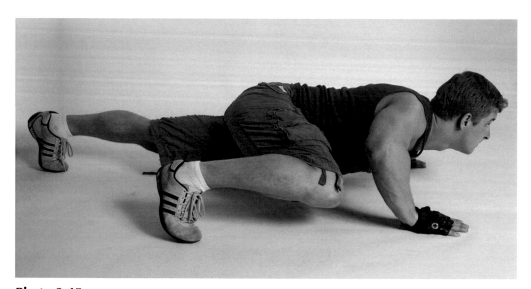

Photo 3.45

Sports applications:
Any sport that utilizes the upper body will benefit, specifically disciplines like rock climbing, swimming, gymnastics, boxing, or martial arts, such as karate.

Come on, warrior, you're not done yet!/progression:

Progression:
Perform the same movement but backward. You will need to start pushing off with the arms as opposed to the legs (in forward Crocodiles) every Crocodile step. That will make the exercise more challenging.

Modification (for persons with shoulder conditions):
Walk forward on all fours, making sure not to bend your arms too far. Or just perform partial push-ups.

Arjuna Tiger Pull/Pulling Band in a Defense Fall

Difficulty level: A

Caution: If you have knee problems, you may be able to perform the exercise modification provided.

Origin: ID

Presenter: Self

Starting position:
Attach a wide, thick band to a high pulley station. Place a mat a few feet away, directly in front of it. Step on the mat with your left shoulder and foot closer to the pulley (left lead). Grasp the band tightly with your right hand. Keep your left arm up in a guard position (see Photo 3.46).

Movement:
While holding the band, suddenly bend your right knee (it should be bending to the outside right) and perform a fall on your right buttock (see Photos 3.47–48). Make sure to contract muscles in the leg and the right buttock as well as the right side to cushion the fall. Let the kinetic momentum rock you back so that the rubber band will be fully stretched. Rock back up the same way you fell initially, using just the right leg to stand up (see Photos 3.49–50). Because you are holding the band, it will be easier for you to come back up. Both the elastic energy in the stretched band and your own

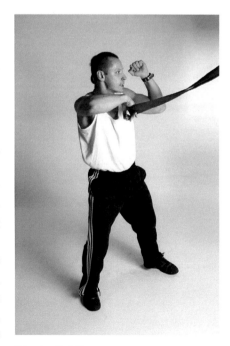

Photo 3.46

body will make it possible for you to quickly spring up. On your way up, forcefully pull the band back (the elbow is out to the side), thus helping yourself up, just as if you were using another person's hand to get up from the floor after falling. Using the kinetic energy generated on going up, and before you lose it, quickly perform a right elbow back strike (your elbow will be raised up and to the side). See Photo 3.51. This will count as one repetition. Start to fall again and perform 15 repetitions. Switch leads and grab the band with your left hand.

Major muscles involved:
In the upper body and trunk, you obviously work the posterior deltoid (rear shoulder), the latissimus dorsi (sides of back), as well as the external obliques (sides), with rectus abdominis (upper abdominals). In the lower body, the quadriceps (front of thigh) are involved. The posterior deltoid is the prime mover for the arm. Muscles in the trunk are assisting in the getting up movement, and the quadriceps serve as the prime movers for the upper body.

Ark's tips:
The key to performing this exercise is speed. Speed is the king! Have you heard that before? You must not be afraid of falling down. Make it a smooth fall. Fall on the right buttock and the inner side of right forearm. Allow the band to slow down the fall and pull you back up. If done correctly, the forceful pulling on the band with the right arm will accelerate your get up.

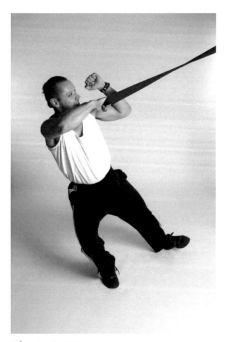

Photo 3.47

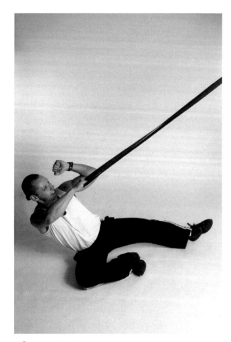

Photo 3.48

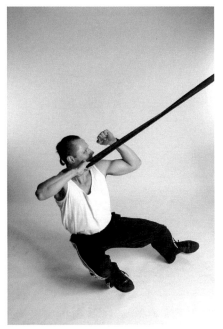

Photo 3.49

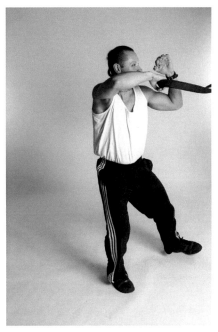

Photo 3.50

Breathing technique:
Relax and inhale as you are falling down. Remember to tighten up the muscles on the right side of your body. Keep contracting them as you start to rock back up and forcefully exhale. The final phase of the exhalation should be done as you complete the quick pull on the band. Next, do a quick inhalation and yet another exhalation when you do the elbow strike.

Sports applications:
Arjuna Tiger Pull will help an athlete in the execution of foundational skills, such as jumping for height or distance, various kicks, or pushing with the lower body. We can mention sports like basketball (shooting), the high jump, bounding, football, soccer, and many kicks in the martial arts. If you are a martial artist, this exercise will improve your dynamic sense of balance, back strikes (e.g., different

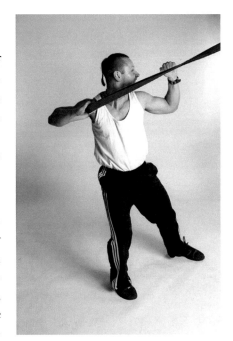

Photo 3.51

forms of back fists), as well as the rearing back part of any punch (which should be done even faster than the actual delivery of a punch).

Come on, warrior, you're not done yet!/progression:

IDP1:
Hold a light dumbbell in your left hand and/or decrease the tension of the band.

Modification (for persons with knee conditions):
See modification exercise for Karate Squats.

     Bhima Pull/One-armed Under Bar Pull-up

     Difficulty level: A

     Caution: If you have back problems, you may be able to perform the exercise modification provided.

     Origin: ID

     Presenter: Warrior Greg

Starting position:
Find a Smith's Squat Machine (it allows you to squat, bench-press, etc., in a controlled manner) and lower the bar so that it is on one of the lowest settings (approximately 2 feet above the floor). After placing a mat under the bar, get under it with your legs bent at the knees. While on your back, grasp the bar with the right hand so that your fist is aligned with the right pectoral muscle (chest). (See Photo 3.52.) If you grasp the bar too far to the right, outside of your body's center line, it will be too difficult to execute the Bhima Pull in good form.

Movement:
Tighten up all of the muscles in the core and lower your body, squeeze the bar tighter, then lift up your hips and torso at the same time. Rely on your right arm to maintain this bridge position. Keep pulling your upper body up until your chest almost touches the bar (see Photos 3.53–57). You should aim at getting both left and right pectoral muscles close to

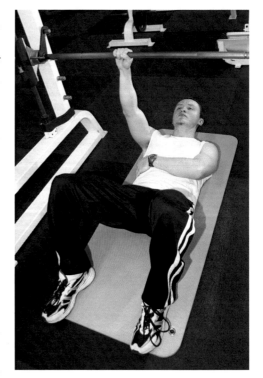

Photo 3.52

the bar, and not just one. Slowly lower yourself to the floor. This counts as one repetition. Perform at least 10 of them and switch arms.

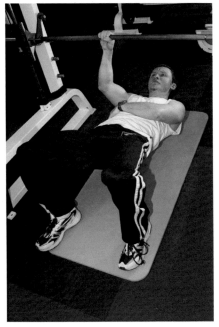

Photo 3.53

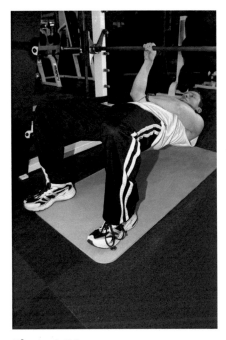

Photo 3.54

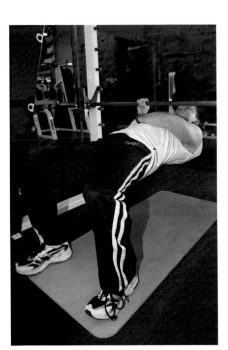

Photo 3.55

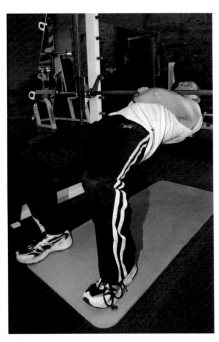

Photo 3.56

Major muscles involved:
In the arm, you work biceps brachii (front of arm), in the trunk, latissimus dorsi (side of back), erector spinae (lower back), in the core, rectus abdominis, as well as external oblique muscles. The prime mover in the Bhima Pull is, of course, the huge latissimus dorsi muscle. Biceps brachii is the assisting mover, and the other muscles perform stabilizing functions. In the lower body, you work the back of the thigh (biceps femoris), as well as the buttocks (gluteus maximus).

Ark's tips:
Contract all the muscles in the body. Do not just work with the upper body. For the Bhima Pull to be done perfectly, you will need to summon the forces of all muscles, such as the legs, butt, lower back, and abs. The total effect of this extreme squeeze will pull you straight up to the bar. Remember that the left and right side of the chest should be aligned so they come near the bar together.

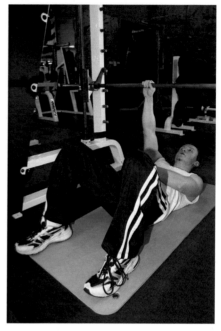

Photo 3.57

Breathing technique:
Hold your breath until you are close to the bar. Once you get there, quickly exhale and inhale on your way down to the mat.

Sports applications:
Bhima Pull will prove effective for all those who practice rowing sports, tennis, gymnastics, swimming (different strokes), etc.

Come on, warrior, you're not done yet!/progression:

IDP1:
Straighten out your legs and perform the Bhima Pull.

Modification (for extension-biased persons[24]):
Perform a double grip Under Bar Pull-up.

    One-legged Squat

    Difficulty level: S

    Caution: If you have knee problems, you may be able to perform the exercise modification provided.

    Origin: K

    Presenter: Self

Starting position:
Find a clear area on a hardwood floor. Commence the exercise by lifting up your left foot. Keep your hands in front of you for balance. See Photo 3.58.

Movement:
Next, bend at the right hip and while keeping your back arched, squat all the way down until you sit on your right heel (see Photos 3.59–61 for the side view). Without relaxing your muscles much, contract muscles in the legs and the core harder and push yourself up. Push from the heel and core. Do at least 10 squats for each leg. See Photos 3.62–64 for a front view of the pushing-up portion.

Major muscles involved:
Muscles such as the front and back of the thigh (quadriceps and hamstring group) do the majority of the work. Gluteus maximus (butt) is also active as an assisting muscle. Other muscles in the leg, such as the soleus in the calf, are assisting the larger

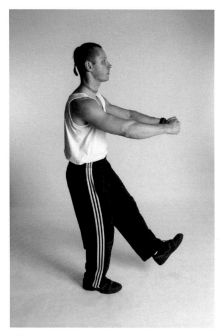

Photo 3.58

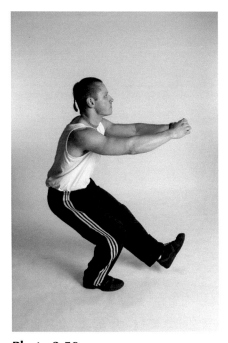

Photo 3.59

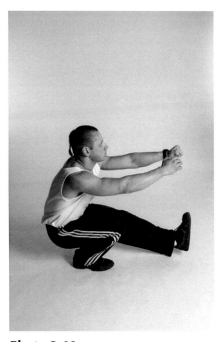

Photo 3.60

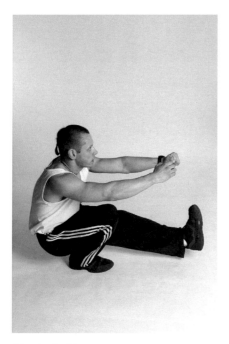

Photo 3.61

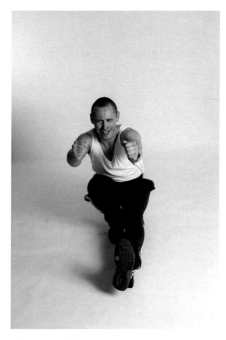

Photo 3.62

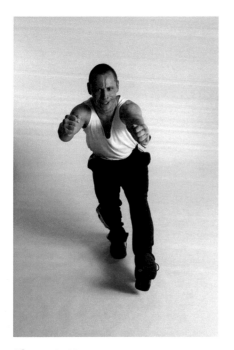

Photo 3.63

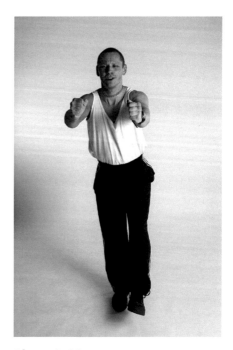

Photo 3.64

muscles in the upper leg to execute the squat. Lower back (erector spinae) and abdominal muscles (rectus abdominis) work as well to aid primarily in the stabilization and balancing of the body throughout the movement.

Ark's tips:
It is essential to shift your weight to the heel and keep your hands in front. Otherwise, you will lose your balance easily. Look straight ahead and visualize yourself doing the squat. It may even be better to stand in front of a mirror and watch your form when performing this difficult exercise. Your back will round at the end of the squat, but you should attempt to keep it arched for as long as you can.

Breathing technique:
Inhale as you squat down and exhale as you push yourself up.

Sports applications:
The One-legged Squat will help a warrior immensely in various kicking actions, skipping, leaping, or pushing with the lower body. More specifically, you will improve your squat jumps, front kicks in karate, front kicks in soccer, kicks in football, running, and standing long jumps, bonding, etc.

Come on, warrior, you're not done yet!/progression:

Progression:
Do the squat on an unstable surface, such as a Bosu ball (rounded half ball). Maintain a steady medium tempo.

Modification (for persons with knee conditions):
Perform partial squats as in the exercise modification for Karna's Fall.

Excellent, now repeat this twice more and record your completion time!

Cooldown. Walk around for a minute and perform stretches for the muscles worked during the training session, such as front and rear shoulders, triceps (back of arm), chest, sides of back, abdominals, legs (both front thigh and back of thigh), etc.

Ending meditation:
Same as for the Beginner Krishna Warrior Fitness Program.

Word of instruction:
Congratulations! You have just completed the third workout plan. Are you feeling THE POWER? Continue with it for the next 6 weeks, three times a week, each time trying to better your form and take less rest. Keep writing down your completion times on your Personal Record Sheet (see Chapter 5). On other days, engage yourself in jogging, any sports of your liking, or skill training that you may need for your specific discipline (football or soccer practice, performing kata or forms in karate). Continue eating in accordance with your body type 7 days a week. Make sure to take 1 day of complete rest. At the end of the

sixth week, you can repeat the whole program as indicated in the Final Assignments section below.

FINAL ASSIGNMENTS

1. (Required) Perform a fitness assessment on yourself, or have someone do it for you. See how much fat weight you've lost and how many pounds of lean muscle you've gained. By now, you should be a fully fledged Krishna warrior and have attained to your fitness goal.

2. (Required) If you gained muscle and lost body fat, you will need to increase your protein intake to keep making gains (increase strength, power, etc.) and burn more fat. If you are a competitive athlete, you should try to apply protein recommendations that your body type requires (see Chapter 4), as well as required supplements (e.g., CoQ10, L-glutamine, etc.).

3. (Optional) If you like the variety and intensity of the exercises and you would like to make further progress, you should repeat all three mesocycles using progressions that were included at the end of each exercise. This time, you can shorten each mesocycle to 3 or even 2 weeks.

Arsenal Two

Gaining

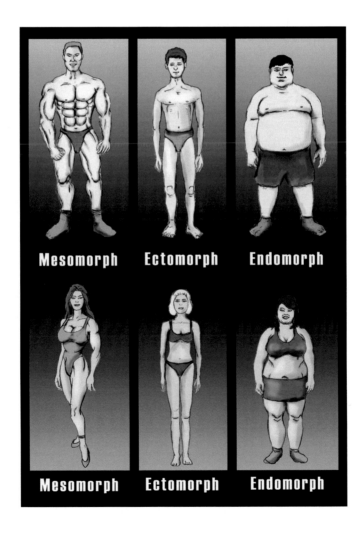

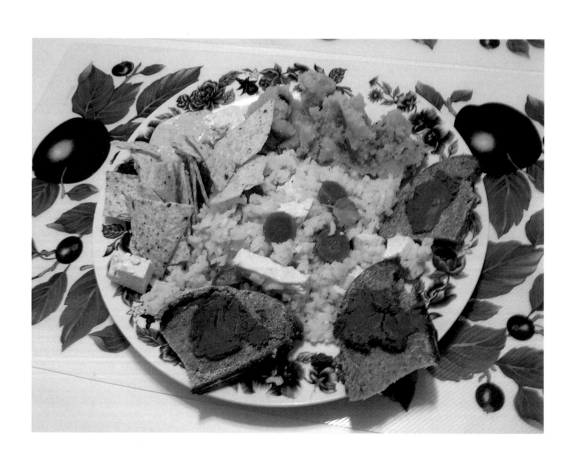

Chapter IV

Nutritional Planning for a Krishna Warrior

Krishna warrior's approach to nutrition is holistic. We take care of our body, mind, and spirit. We look at the big perspective. We worry less about calories, grams, or points. The ancient medical scriptures of India, China, and Greece give such a perspective.

For example, one of the ancient fathers of medicine, Hippocrates, said that "It appears to me necessary to every physician to be skilled in nature and to strive to know, if he would wish to perform his duties, what man is in relation to the articles of food and drink and to his other occupations and what are the effects of each of them on everyone. Whoever does not know what effect these things produce upon a man cannot know the consequences which result from them. Whoever pays no attention to these things . . . how can he understand the diseases which befall man? For by every one of these things a man is affected and changed this way and that, and the whole of his life is subject to them—whether in health, convalescence, or disease" (quoted in Danavir 209).

In the chapter to follow, I will present simplified parts of Indian or Ayurvedic medicine as regards to body types, along with some other natural perspectives such as Chinese medicine.

SEEING THE BIG PICTURE

Ayurveda literally means "the science of life and longevity." It teaches that the body is a machine made of the same elements as other things in nature. Let me explain. When you really break the body down, it is just water, earth, fire, ether, and air. The whole material energy is made up of the same basic elements, just like the whole science of mathematics is based on numbers from 1 to 9, or any book you pick up on the shelf is made up of 24 letters, the alphabet. The difference is in the level of science or the level of writing. Similarly, plants, vegetables, animals, etc., consist of the same basic elements as human bodies. The only difference is the structural arrangement and concentration of the elements.

The five elements that are present in our body are in a constant flux that is directed toward entropy, or dissipation. The five elements of our body are vibrating for a certain amount of time and thereafter need to leave their present structure to become free and join the universal elements of water, earth, fire, etc. Smaller structures, or parts, want to join bigger parts. This is one of the universal laws we ought to know about.

When we eat, we supply and replenish our bodies with a certain amount of the five elements so the force of the bodily machine increases, or remains stable. If we don't provide those elements, then the body becomes depleted and the machine of the body breaks down.

Consequently, the spirit soul, which is of a completely different, immaterial nature, will relinquish the ruined structure and look for a different shelter. It is much like after driving a car for some time. You need to supply it with petroleum, change the oil, check the tires, unless you want it to break down on the road.

YOUR BODY TYPE

The key to healthy nutrition and, therefore, living, is knowing your body type. A body type denotes your particular physical structure (bones, muscles, etc.), as well as your particular metabolic functioning (e.g., how fast you digest food and how each food effects your body). It is just like a mechanic knowing a particular car. Each of us has a slightly different concentration of the five elements, both in subtle (mental) state and gross (physical) state.

Similarly, different species of vegetables, fruits, grains, etc., have different concentrations of the five elements. It is just like knowing that driving a diesel will require a different fuel than driving a Honda. Both are fuels, but each one is for different kinds of cars. Of course, this is a crude example, but I think you get the idea. We will first discuss physical aspects of body types, and then their metabolic aspects.

The modern fitness science recognizes body typing at some levels. They are based mainly on the works of Dr. William H. Sheldon, who introduced his theory of somatypes[25] in the 1940s in his *Varieties of Human Physique*. In that book, we can find descriptions of three main body types, or morphological components: ectomorph, mesomorph, and endomorph. An ectomorph has a rather thin, small-framed body with a naturally high metabolism, and finds it difficult to put on muscle weight. A mesomorph has a medium frame, with well-defined musculature, and gains muscle easily. An endomorph has a body with a naturally low metabolism, medium to large frame, and has a tendency to put on fat weight (ISSA 1).

Sheldon's description of body types has become important to much of the literature on exercise and bodybuilding. He describes 76 variations of the three body types. However, the ideas of body types and their corresponding psychological types did not originate with Sheldon.

YOUR PERSONALITY AND BODY TYPE

The physical structure of a body is often related to the person's personality, and Dr. Sheldon briefly presents three personality types (234–36) in his book. They are further elaborated upon in *The Varieties of Human Temperament*. But Plato's *The Republic* and Indian medical scriptures describe similar principles. For example, Ayurvedic body typing categorizations (Pita, Vata, Kapha) and their descriptions, as well as the corresponding personality types closely resemble Dr. Sheldon's presentation. He, himself, mentions Hippocrates, the ancient Greek doctor, who designated two fundamental body types (Sheldon 10). Many French, German, Italian, and English researchers conducted studies and postulated theories about body types, most of which were mentioned in *The Varieties of Human Physique*. One may mention here names such as Halle, de Troisvèvre, Rostan, di Giovanni, Huter, Viola, Kretschmer, etc.

I found that the medical science of Ayurveda renders a very complete description of how to know your body type and how to optimally maintain the body. Knowing your body type and eating in accordance with it greatly affect fat loss, muscle gain, performance, and how you feel. In Dr. Sheldon's work, the bodies' particular food needs according to body type are also mentioned but no conclusive recommendations are made (248–9). But this is exactly what Ayurveda offers.

YOUR NUTRITIONAL BODY TYPE

Your physical body type will affect how you metabolize, or digest, certain foods. Let me give you a simple example. Let's say that I am a tiger, and you start feeding me vegetables! Or, let's say I am an elephant, and you start feeding me some animal flesh. Well, it will take some time before I get used to my new food, or will I be optimally healthy even after getting used to my new food? Tigers, by nature, are carnivores, and their special bodily structure calls for a particular kind of food. Elephants, by nature, are vegetarians.

Dr. William Wolcott, author of *The Metabolic Typing Diet*, provides us with a very comprehensive system of metabolic body typing which utilizes Ayurvedic and Chinese medicine as one of the nine[26] fundamental diagnostic tools to find body types. This results in three basic metabolic types: protein type, carbo type, and mixed type. They roughly correspond to Ayurvedic Vata, Pita, Kapha types, and Sheldon's body types.

Sheldon's focus was on physical measurements of bodies and psychological ramifications of it, whereas, Wolcott's was more on physiological/metabolic processes that occur inside the body without concern for personality, behavior, or physical looks. Whereas Sheldon does not give any nutritional recommendations for body types, Wolcott does give specific guidelines for each body type. Ayurveda, itself, considers physical traits as well as psychological traits of a person and assigns them specific food regimens and lifestyles. Therefore, it is my contention that the ancient and well tested by time Ayurvedic presentation itself will be the most complete and satisfying to the reader.

The first step is to look at the physical and psychological (subtle matter) concentration of the five elements in our bodies. You do that by answering the questions below and collecting your Air, Space, Fire, Water, and Earth points. When you answer the questions, think of your whole life and general tendencies, rather than just recent months or years. Pick only one answer and collect two points for each of the elements.

The questionnaire I provided below is a simplified one[27] and is based on Ayurveda (Lad 18–19). You may use it as an initial guide to finding your physical and psychological body type.

BODY TYPE QUIZ

1. What's your body size?

    a) slim   Air and Space (AS)
    b) medium   Fire and Water (FW)
    c) large   Earth and Water (EW)

2. If you don't exercise and eat your normal food, what weight does your body tend toward?

    a) low   AS
    b) medium   FW
    c) overweight   EW

3. How is your digestion?

    a) irregular, gas forming   AS
    b) quick, causes burning   FW
    c) slow, may form mucus   EW

4. Is your skin ...

    a) dry, cold, rough   AS
    b) smooth, oily, warm   FW
    c) thick, oily, cool, white   EW

5. Is your hair ...

    a) thin, brittle   AS
    d) straight, oily, red, or bald   FW
    c) thick, oily, curly   EW

6. Are your teeth ...

    a) protruding, big, thin gums   AS
    b) medium, tender gums   FW
    c) white, strong gums   EW

7. Are your eyes ...

    a) small, dry, active, black, nervous   AS
    b) sharp, bright, gray, green   FW
    c) big, blue, calm   EW

8. Is your nose ...

    a) Uneven   AS
    b) long, pointed, red nose tip   FW
    c) short, rounded   EW

9. Are your nails ...

    a) dry, rough, brittle   AS
    b) sharp, flexible, pink   FW
    c) thick, oily, smooth   EW

10. Are your lips ...
   a) dry, cracked   AS
   b) red, inflamed   FW
   c) smooth, oily   EW

11. Are your cheeks ...
   a) sunken   AS
   b) smooth, flat   FW
   c) rounded, plump   EW

12. Is your chin ...
   a) thin, angular   AS
   b) tapering   FW
   c) rounded   EW

13. Your neck is ...
   a) thin, tall   AS
   b) medium   FW
   c) big   EW

14. Is your chest ...
   a) flat, sunken   AS
   b) medium   FW
   c) expanded, round   EW

15. Is your stomach ...
   a) thin, sunken   AS
   b) medium   FW
   c) big, potbellied   EW

16. Are your hips ...
   a) slender, thin   AS
   b) medium   FW
   c) heavy, big   EW

17. Are your joints ...
   a) cold, cracking   AS
   b) moderate   FW
   c) large, lubricated   EW

18. What foods do you prefer?
   a) sweet, sour, salty   AS
   b) sweet, bitter, astringent (e.g., beans)   FW
   c) bitter, pungent, astringent   EW

19. How is your appetite?
    a) irregular, small   AS
    b) strong   FW
    c) slow but steady   EW

20. How thirsty do you get throughout the day?
    a) it varies   AS
    b) always thirsty   FW
    c) not very thirsty   EW

21. How would you rate your daily physical activity?
    a) I am hyperactive   AS
    b) Moderate   FW
    c) I like to be sedentary   EW

22. How would you rate your normal mental activity?
    a) I am always active   AS
    b) I am in the middle   FW
    c) Slow   EW

23. How would you describe your emotional tendencies?
    a) flexible, anxiety, fear, uncertainty   AS
    b) anger, hate, jealous, determined   FW
    c) calm, greedy, attached to things   EW

24. How strong is your resolve or discipline?
    a) changeable   AS
    b) intense, extreme   FW
    c) consistent, mellow   EW

25. How is your intellectual activity?
    a) react fast but often incorrectly   AS
    b) accurate reaction or response   FW
    c) slow but exact response   EW

26. How is your memory?
    a) recent good, remote not so good   AS
    b) good recollection of past and present   FW
    c) slow recollection but sustained   EW

27. How is your sleeping pattern?
    a) broken up, sleeplessness   AS
    b) kind of short but sound   FW
    c) deep, prolonged   EW

28. How do you talk?

    a) fast, unclear   AS

    b) medium, penetrating, sharp   FW

    c) slow, monotonous   EW

Now that you collected your points, add them up and see how many of each element you got. For example, if you pick answer "C" to question 28, you collect one Earth point and one Water point.

Air and Space elements form an Ectomorph (Vata) body type, Fire and Water form a Mesomorph (Pita), and Earth and Water form an Endomorph (Kapha) body type. So if you got mostly Airs and Spaces, you are a predominantly Ectomorph body type, both physiologically and psychologically. If your points come mostly from Fire and Water elements, you can identify your body type as Mesomorph. And let's say that your second biggest score came from Air and Space elements. That would mean that your second predominant type is Ectomorph.

Just so you know, every one of us has all of the five elements in the body, but here we are trying to determine a predominance of certain elements. There certainly are possibilities of dual body types. For example, you may collect an almost equal amount of Airs and Fires. So you can identify your body as half Ectomorph and half Mesomorph. There are also trios that have an equal amount of AS, FW, and EW. But that is rare.

The second step is to find out which foods have higher concentrations of the elements that you naturally have less of. So here I provide a simplified list that is by no means exhaustive, also based on the Ayurveda (Lad 82–96), which mentions foods that have a balancing effect on your particular body type. Basically, you consume more of the foods that contain the elements you lack and less of the foods that contain an ample amount of elements you possess.

So check your score, and then align yourself with one predominant body type. Next, go to the charts and see what's there for your body type. Do not worry as much about glycemic index[28] of the foods, calories, and grams. Try to feel which foods make you feel energized and satisfied in body and mind.

ECTOMORPH BALANCING FOODS (ETHER AND SPACE PREDOMINANT)

Fruit:

Consume most sweet fruits, such as:

apples (cooked), applesauce, avocados, bananas, berries, coconuts, grapes, grapefruit, lemons, mangos, melons, oranges, papaya, peaches, pineapples, plums, raisins, strawberries

Avoid dried fruits

Vegetables:

Consume cooked vegetables, such as:

asparagus, carrots, green beans, leeks, okra, black olives, parsnip, peas, sweet potatoes, pumpkins, summer and winter squash, watercress, zucchini

Avoid frozen, raw, or dried vegetables

Grains: Durham flour, cooked oats, pancakes, quinoa, all types of rice, sprouted wheat, Essene bread, wheat

Avoid:
barley; bread with yeast; buckwheat; dried, puffed cereals; corn; crackers; granola; muesli; rye

Legumes:
Consume mung beans

Avoid:
most beans

Dairy:
Consume most dairy products, such as butter, soft cheese, cottage cheese, cow's milk, clarified butter (Ghee), goat's milk

Avoid:
powdered milk, plain and frozen yogurt

Animal foods:
Consume chicken (dark meat), duck, eggs, freshwater or sea fish, salmon, sardines, other seafood, shrimp

Avoid:
beef, lamb, pork, venison, white turkey

Condiments:
Consume kelp, ketchup, lemons, lime pickles, mayonnaise, mustard, pickles, salt, scallions, seaweed, tamari, vinegar

Avoid:
chocolate, horseradish

Nuts:
all are good for you

Seeds:
Consume chia, flax, pumpkin, sesame, sunflower, tahini

Avoid:
popcorn

Oils:
Consume most oils

Avoid:
flaxseed

Beverages:
Consume almond milk, aloe vera juice, apple cider, carrot juice, chai (hot), lemonade, rice milk, sour juices

Avoid:
apple juice, black tea, caffeinated drinks, carbonated drinks, chocolate milk, coffee, cold dairy drinks, cranberry juice, iced tea, mixed vegetable juice, pomegranate juice, V-8, soy milk

Sweeteners:
Consume fructose, fruit juice concentrates, raw and unprocessed honey, molasses, rice syrup, sucanat, turbinado

Avoid:
white sugar

Supplements:
Consume bee pollen, amino acids, calcium, copper, iron, magnesium, zinc, spirulina, blue-green algae, vitamins A, B complex, C, D, E

Avoid:
barley green, brewer's yeast

MESOMORPH BALANCING FOODS (FIRE AND WATER PREDOMINANT)

Fruit:
Consume most sweet fruit, such as:
apples, applesauce, avocados, berries, coconuts, grapes (red, purple), mangos, melons, oranges, peaches, pineapples, plums, raisins, watermelons

Avoid sour fruits

Vegetables:
Consume sweet and bitter vegetables, such as:
artichokes, asparagus, bitter melons, broccoli, Brussels sprouts, cabbages, cooked carrots, cauliflower, celery, cucumbers, leafy greens, lettuce, mushrooms, okra, black olives, parsley, peas, sweet peppers, sweet potatoes, white potatoes, winter and summer squash, wheatgrass sprouts, zucchini

Avoid:
pungent vegetables such as raw beets, garlic, green chilies, horseradish, mustard greens, green olives, raw onions, tomatoes, raw spinach

Grains:
Consume amaranth, barley, dry cereal, couscous, crackers, Durham flour, granola, oat bran, cooked oats, pancakes, pasta, white and wild rice, rice cakes, spelt, Essene bread, tapioca, wheat, wheat bran

Avoid:
Bread with yeast, buckwheat, corn, dry oats, millet, quinoa, brown rice, rye

Legumes:
Consume most beans

Avoid:
miso, soy sauce, soy sausage

Dairy:
Consume unsalted butter; unsalted, soft cheese; cottage cheese; cow's milk; clarified butter (Ghee); goat's milk; ice cream

Avoid:
salted butter, buttermilk, hard-aged cheese, sour cream, plain or frozen yogurt

Animal foods:
Consume chicken (white), egg whites, freshwater fish, white turkey, venison

Avoid:
all others such as beef, dark chicken, lamb, pork, salmon, tuna, fish (sea), dark turkey

Condiments:
Consume coriander, sprouts

Avoid:
chili pepper, chocolate, horseradish, ketchup, mustard, lemon, lime pickle, mayonnaise, salt, scallions, seaweed, soy sauce, vinegar

Nuts:
Consume almonds soaked in purified water, coconut

Avoid:
almonds with skin, cashews, filberts, hazelnuts, Macademia nuts, peanuts, walnuts

Seeds:
Consume flax, sunflower

Avoid:
chia, sesame, tahini

Oils:
Consume sunflower, ghee (clarified butter), olive, soy, flaxseed, walnut

Avoid:
almond, corn, safflower, sesame

Beverages:
Consume almond milk, aloe vera juice, apple juice, black tea, carob, cool dairy drinks, grain "coffee," grape juice, mango juice, mixed vegetable juice, peach nectar

Avoid:

apple cider, caffeinated drinks, carbonated drinks, carrot juice, chocolate milk, coffee, cranberry juice, grapefruit juice, iced tea, lemonade, mixed vegetable juice, sour juices (pineapple), tomato juice, V-8 juice

Sweeteners:

Consume barley malt, fructose, fruit juice concentrates, maple syrup, rice syrup, sucanat, turbinado

Avoid:

honey, molasses, white sugar

Supplements:

Consume aloe vera juice, barley green, brewer's yeast, calcium, magnesium, zinc, spirulina, blue-green algae, vitamins D, E

Avoid:

amino acids, copper, iron, vitamins A, B complex, C

ENDOMORPH BALANCING FOODS (EARTH AND WATER PREDOMINANT)

Fruit:

Consume most astringent fruits, such as:

Apples, applesauce, apricots, berries, cherries, cranberries, pears, persimmons, pomegranates, prunes, raisins

Avoid sweet and sour fruits, such as:

avocados, bananas, coconuts, dates, grapefruit, kiwi, melons, oranges, papayas, pineapples, plums, rhubarb, watermelons

Vegetables:

Consume pungent and bitter vegetables, such as:

artichokes, asparagus, beets, broccoli, cabbages, carrots, cauliflower, celery, eggplant, garlic, green beans, green chilies, horseradish, kale, leafy greens, leeks, lettuce, mushrooms, okra, onions, parsley, white potatoes, spinach, sprouts, tomatoes (cooked), turnips, watercress, wheatgrass, sprouts

Avoid sweet and juicy vegetables:

cucumbers, olives, sweet potatoes, pumpkin, winter squash, raw tomatoes, zucchini

Grains:

Consume barley, buckwheat, cereal (dry, puffed), couscous, crackers, granola, millet, muesli, oat bran, dry oats, polenta, rye, Essene bread, tapioca, wheat bran

Avoid:

bread with yeast, cooked oats, pancakes, rice, wheat

Legumes:
Consume Adzuki beans, black beans, chickpeas, lentils (red, brown), lima beans, navy beans, peas (dried), soy milk, split peas, tempeh, white beans

Avoid:
kidney beans, soybeans, soy cheese, soy flower, soy powder, soy sauce, tofu (cold), miso

Dairy:
Consume cottage cheese from skimmed goat's milk, goat's milk (skim), diluted yogurt

Avoid:
butter, cheese, cow's milk, ice cream, sour cream, yogurt (plain and frozen)

Animal foods:
Consume chicken (white), duck, eggs, freshwater fish, rabbit, shrimp, white turkey, venison

Avoid:
beef, buffalo, dark chicken, duck, fish (sea), lamb, pork, sardines, turkey (dark)

Condiments:
Consume black pepper, chili pepper, horseradish, mustard, scallions, sprouts

Avoid:
chocolate, kelp, lime, lime pickle, mayonnaise, pickles, salt, soy sauce, tamari, vinegar

Nuts:
Avoid all nuts

Seeds:
Consume chia, popcorn (no salt or butter)

Avoid:
sesame, tahini

Oils:
Consume corn, sesame, sunflower, ghee (clarified butter), almond

Avoid:
coconut, olive, primrose, safflower, sesame, soy, walnut

Beverages:
Consume aloe vera juice, apple cider, black tea, carob, carrot juice, cherry juice, cranberry juice, grape juice, mango juice, peach nectar, pomegranate juice, prune juice, soy milk (hot and spiced)

Avoid:
almond milk, caffeinated drinks, carbonated drinks, chocolate milk, coffee, cold dairy drinks, grapefruit juice, iced tea, icy cold drinks, orange juice, rice milk, V-8 juice, soy milk (cold), tomato juice

Sweeteners:
Consume fruit juice concentrates, raw and unprocessed honey

Avoid:
fructose, maple syrup, molasses, rice syrup, turbinado, white sugar

Supplements:
Consume aloe vera juice, amino acids, barley green, brewer's yeast, copper, calcium, iron, magnesium, zinc, spirulina, blue-green algae, vitamins A, B, C, D, E.

Avoid:
potassium

I also recommend you make a list of foods that you absolutely hate, that you are indifferent to, and that you absolutely love. Try not to look at ready-made items, such as a fruit smoothies, shakes, or pizzas, but at more basic articles, such as cheese, milk, pineapple, rice, cauliflower, etc. Keep things simple. Start from the basics and arrive at good principles of healthy eating. Your likes or dislikes, which may change over time, often show your natural or acquired tendencies (not always healthy). Such tendencies often have to do with your body type.

EATING AT THE RIGHT TIME—SOLAR NUTRITION

A Krishna warrior not only eats the right kind of food for his body type, but he or she also eats it at the best time. Chinese culture has a lot to offer in terms of knowledge such as health and natural medicine. For example, solar nutrition, which is based on the ancient Chinese medical books, is a very gentle and natural approach that enhances our mental and physical health.

Solar nutrition also synthesizes the latest advances in chronobiology with the fundamental premises of acupuncture and the ancient Chinese knowledge of the cosmology of the human body. Acupuncture postulates that different meridians form circuit systems in the body, with specific organs, glands, tissues, muscles, and nervous systems on individual circuits, and that these circuits function differently, at different times of the day, determined by the position of the sun relative to the earth (eatsolar.com).

Solar nutrition teaches us how to eat foods at specific times based on the body organ's optimum nutrient utilization (Harting 7). This approach is designed to maximize the utilization and assimilation of the sun's energy from food, release cellular trauma, and optimize health and vitality. Foods have different nutritional values at different times of the day. The organs of the body function on a schedule, and the pH (level of acidity) of digestive fluid changes throughout the day (eatsolar.com).

When you eat certain foods at certain times of the day, it ensures that food nutrients are aligned with the nutritional needs of the body, providing complete digestion of the proteins, carbohydrates, fats, vitamins, and minerals (eatsolar.com).

It works when the plants capture the sun's energy via photosynthesis, and our bodies utilize this energy by digesting the plants as food. By eating certain foods at certain times of the day, we can maximize our assimilation of solar energy from our food. The human body also has the ability to directly absorb solar power. The hypothalamus, the pineal gland, and the retina of the eye trap light like a plant and convert it to energy (eatsolar.com).

Below, I provide simplified lists of morning, afternoon, and evening foods, regardless of your body type (Eatsolar.com; Harting, 219–233).

MORNING FOODS
MIDNIGHT TO NOON—BEST BETWEEN 7 A.M.–9 A.M.

NUTS
almonds
apricot kernels
brazil
carob
cashews, roasted
coconut
filbert
hazel
macadamia
pecans
pine nuts

BEANS
cocoa
dark chocolate

SWEETENERS
honey
maple syrup

FRUITS
apples
apricots
avocados
bananas
cherries
coconuts
dates
figs
guavas
kiwi
mangos
nectarines
olives
papayas
pears
persimmons
plaintains
plums
pomegranates

prunes
tamarind

CITRUS FRUITS
(Eat alone, best
around 10:00 a.m.)
grapefruit
kumquats
lemons
limes
oranges
tangerines

OILS
almond
apricot
avocado
coconut cream
olive
walnut

MIDDAY FOODS
NOON TO 6:00 P.M.

VEGETABLES
artichokes (globe)
beans (dried or fresh)
bitter melon
broccoli
Brussels sprouts
cabbage
cauliflower
celery
cereals
corn
cucumber
eggplant
endive
escarole
grains
herbs
lettuce
okra
parsley
peppers, hot
(cayenne only)
peppers, sweet
(bell, yellow banana)
pumpkin
spinach
sprouts (all kinds)
squash
tomatoes
water cress

FRUITS
blackberries
blueberries
boysenberries
cranberries
dewberries
grapes
raisins
raspberries
strawberries

SEEDS
caraway
flax
pumpkin
sesame
sunflower

OILS
ghee (clarified butter)
safflower
sesame
soy
sunflower
wheat germ

SWEETENERS
brown sugar
honey
molasses
rice syrup

BREADS
all kinds if natural

CHEESES
all kinds if natural

MILK, SOURED
buttermilk
yogurt

MEATS
beef
fowl
lamb
pork
venison

MELONS (best eaten between 3:00–5:00 p.m. and alone)
cantaloupes
casaba
honeydews
watermelons

NIGHT FOODS
6:00 P.M.–9:00 P.M.

SEAFOOD
abalone
all fish except trout
lobster
scallop
shrimp

EGGS

TOFU

NUTS
peanuts

ALGAE

VEGETABLES
artichoke hearts
asparagus

bamboo shoots
beets
celery root
dulce
garlic
ginger root
kelp
leeks
lotus root
mushrooms
onions
parsnips
potatoes
radishes
rutabagas
scallions
sea cucumber
sweet potatoes
turnip

water chestnuts
yams

FRUITS
pineapples
prickly pear cactus

OILS
garlic oil
ghee (clarified butter)
peanut oil

NEUTRAL FOODS
brown rice

basmati brown rice

clarified butter (ghee)

ice cream (made from 100 percent whole cream)

olive oil

probiotics

whole cream

FOOD AND MENTAL HEALTH

In *Nutrition and Your Mind*, Dr. George Watson, a renown clinical psychologist, said that "when one knows nothing of nutrition and eats merely from ignorance, habit, and learned prejudices, there is a steady decrease in physical—and often mental—performance as the years of youth go by (65)." He further informs us that "what one eats, digests, and assimilates provides the energy-producing nutrients that the bloodstream carries to the brain. . .

Any interference with the nutritional supply lines or with the energy-producing systems of the brain results in impaired functioning, which then may be called poor mental health (15)."

Watson developed a nutritional system based on a person's metabolic differences, specifically on the rate at which cells convert nutrients into energy. In other words, some people digest food quickly and some slowly.[29] He further discovered that by prescribing specific foods and nutrients to patients, their clinical problems were cured (Mercola 36).

WHAT ARE YOU EATING FOR?

The only two options for a Krishna warrior are: eating for optimum health or maximum performance. Since you already picked up this book and are reading it, I assume that you do not plan on just eating to survive, but at least to achieve optimal health, or even for maximum performance. But most of the diets eaten by the general population can be categorized as "eating for survival."

The Recommended Daily Allowances or Recommended Daily Intakes are based on population averages and are supposed to determine the national health average, not individual health average (Gastelu and Hatfield 12). Many progressive nutritionists confirm what the ancient medical scriptures already stated, namely, that our bodies need whole, fresh foods for optimal well-being. Why? Because whole foods simply have more life force and nutrients that our bodies need.

The medical scriptures of Ayurveda (Lad 82, 96) teach that ectomorphs' and mesomorphs' nutrition should ideally consist of 50 percent body-type-specific (bts) (see body type food charts above) whole grains, 20 percent body-type-specific protein, and 20–30 percent body-type-specific fresh vegetables (optional 10 percent for fresh fruit). Endomorphs should eat 30–40 percent bts whole grains, 20 percent bts protein, 40–50 percent bts fresh vegetables (optional 10 percent for fresh or dried fruit).

Eating for performance is yet another level of eating. Although the *Krishna Warrior Fitness Challenge* focuses on the optimum health view of nutrition, which the Ayurveda presents, some athletes who read the book might benefit from additional knowledge on eating for specific performance needs based on their sports discipline and/or body type. Not that this may necessarily correlate with eating for optimum well-being of the body, mind, and spirit.

If you are a predominant ectomorph and would like to train for muscle and strength gain, or even a specific sport discipline (football, wrestling), you will need more protein than other body types (since it is hard for you to put on muscle weight) and a moderate amount of fat (since your tendency is to stay lean). Keep the carbohydrate-to-protein ratio of 1:2. High glycemic carbohydrates are great for you! But use carbohydrates with a low glycemic index, such as brown rice, whole barley, apples, berries, oranges, and yogurt. Consume approximately 2 grams of protein and 4 grams of carbohydrates per pound of body weight. Eat six times a day, if not more (1 Underhill 1–2).

If you are a predominant mesomorph and would like to train for muscle and strength gain, you will need about 1.5 grams of protein per pound of body weight. The protein-to-carbohydrate ratio should be about 3:4 (300 g protein, 400 g carbs). As with the ectomorph, your carbohydrates should come mostly from the low glycemic group. However, you do not need them as much as the ectomorph. Eat a little more fat (which should naturally be present with your protein foods such as eggs, milk, cottage cheese) and your body will use it as energy. Consume six meals per day (2 Underhill 2).

If you are a predominant endomorph and would like to train for muscle gain and fat loss, you will need about 1.25 grams of protein per pound of body weight, which is less than the requirement for mesos and ectos. You will need more aerobic training than other body types to lean out. As in the case of ectomorphs and mesomorphs, your carbohydrates should come mostly from the low glycemic group. Eat a little more fat (which should naturally be present with your protein foods such as yogurt, eggs) and your body will use it as energy. Consume six meals per day (G 3–4).

THE CONCEPT OF PURINE FOODS

The name "purine" was invented by a German chemist Emil Fischer in the late nineteenth century. Fischer synthesized it from uric acid for the first time in 1899. A purine is an organic compound found in nature that makes up one of the two groups of nitrogenous bases. These nitrogenous bases, in turn, make up a crucial part of DNA, RNA, and the framework for the universal genetic code. Purines also play an important role in a number of other molecules such as ATP, GTP, Coenzyme A, etc. Examples of notable purines are adenine, guanine, hypoxanthine, xanthine, theobromine, caffeine, uric acid, and isoguanine. The purine synthesized by Emil Fischer does not occur in nature ("Foods with High Purine" 1).

One of the important determinations Dr. Wolcott makes in *The Metabolic Typing Diet* is that certain body types such as protein types must eat high-purine foods in order to stay in optimum health. Foods high in purines are basically meats and meat products, such as organ meats, sweetbreads, anchovies, sardines, herring, mackerel, scallops, etc. Moderate amounts of purines are contained in beef, pork, poultry, other seafood, and some vegetables, such as asparagus, cauliflower, spinach, mushrooms, green peas, beans, oatmeal, wheat bran, and wheat germ. Plant-based foods usually have a low purine content ("Foods with High Purine" 2).

It is my contention that if you are a protein type, you will function at optimal health consuming ample amounts of protein foods that have medium or low purine content. Let me explain. Purine does not exactly mean protein. A more precise proxy for purine is muscle (Saag and Choi 5). A protein-type person, by definition, does need protein but not necessarily from high-purine sources.

Research shows that out of 22 amino acids present in proteins, only eight must be supplied in ready-to-use form from food sources in order for the human body to synthesize necessary muscle protein (for more information on this, see Appendix A). All the other amino acids can be created from other individual nutrients. Perfect examples of complete low-puine proteins are raw milk and almond milk.

In a study, high consumption of meat and seafood were linked to an elevated risk of gout onset (41 percent and 50 percent, respectively). On the other hand, high consumption of dairy products, which are rich in protein but low in purines, was associated with a 44 percent decrease in the incidence of gout disease. Furthermore, consumption of vegetables that had a medium purine content, or a high-protein diet per se, were not significantly correlated with gout disease (Saag 5).

The production of uric acid increases by consuming acidifying foods, and especially any form of meat. On the other hand, most fruits, vegetables, and dairy products (in raw form) are alkaline, or only slightly acidifying. An eminent Danish nutritionist Mikkel Hindhede has said that a low-protein vegetable diet is conducive to alkaline blood while a diet high in protein from meat will form acid, thus increasing acidity of the blood (Danavir 235). Russell Chittenden, often regarded as the "father of American biochemistry," who led the country's first biochemistry department at Yale University, shared these findings about purine protein consumption: "With protein foods . . . when oxidized, they yield a row of crystalline nitrogenous products which ultimately pass out of the body through the kidneys. These nitrogen-based protein by-products frequently spoken of as toxins float about through the body and may exercise more or less of a deleterious influence upon the system (Danavir 236)."

CAN YOU CHANGE YOUR BODY TYPE?

Many clients ask me the question: "If I train hard enough, will I look like so-and-so?" My answer to them is, "Rest assured, if you train smart and hard, you will look and feel your best." Your fitness level will be determined mostly by training smart and hard, whereas your physique will change in the aspects of body fat loss and muscular gain. You see, your muscle can either increase in size or decrease. In this way, it is like a balloon. The shape of the muscle will vary depending on your body type, and not on your training. The visibility of the muscle (tone) will depend on how much fat you lose, and that is directly related to proper nutrition. Dr. Sheldon makes an interesting statement in this regard: "In order for the somatotype to change, the skeleton must change, as well as the shape of the head, the bony structure of the face, the neck, wrists, ankles, calves, and forearms, and the relations of stature to measurements made at places where fat does not accumulate. The deposit or removal of fat does not change the somatotype, for it does not change significantly any of the measurements except those where the fat is deposited (Sheldon 221)."

BODY TYPE–BASED DAILY SCHEDULE

Next, we can go back to the "optimum well-being" principle and learn what a good daily schedule would be for your body type (Tiwari 187–89; Lad 58–63).

ECTOMORPH

6:00 a.m. Wake up and rise promptly. Take a warm shower. Drink a glass of warm to hot water (not from the tap!). Perform calming activities for your mind and spirit, such as prayer, meditation, yoga.

8:00 a.m. Eat breakfast.

10:00 a.m.–2:00 p.m. work time.

11:00 a.m.–noon. Lunch and rest time.

12:00 p.m.–5:00 p.m. more work time. Squeezing in a 30-minute strength workout would be great!

6:00–7:00 p.m. Dinner.

7:00–10:00 p.m. Walk or perform some other relaxing activities, such as meditation or prayer.

10:00 p.m. Bedtime.

MESOMORPH

5:30 a.m. Wake up and rise promptly. Take a cool shower. Drink a glass of lukewarm water (not from the tap!). Perform calming activities for mind and spirit, such as prayer, meditation, or yoga. You could do a 30-minute run, too.

7:30 a.m. Eat breakfast.

10:00 a.m.–2:00 p.m. Work time. This is a good time to do your strength workout.

11:00 a.m.–noon. Lunch and rest time.

12:00–6:00 p.m. More work time.

7:00 p.m. Dinner.

7:00–10:00 p.m. Take a long walk, or perform some other relaxing activities such as meditation or reading.

10:00–11:00 p.m. Bedtime.

ENDOMORPH

4:30 a.m. Wake up and rise promptly. Take a warm shower. Drink a glass of warm to hot water (not from the tap!). Perform calming activities for mind and spirit, such as prayer, meditation, or yoga. You can run for 30 minutes or do strength training.

7:00 a.m. Eat breakfast.

10:00 a.m.–2:00 p.m. Work time.

Noon–1:00 p.m. Lunch.

1:00–5:00 p.m. More work time.

7:00–8:00 p.m. Dinner.

8:00–10:00 p.m. Engage in stimulating activities (don't just nap or watch TV!), such as light exercises or yoga.

11:00–midnight. Prayer, meditation, bedtime.

BEWARE OF WEIGHT LOSS DIETS

First of all, some of the fad diets out there may not provide you with enough calories even to function properly at home and work, let alone to exercise five to six times a week. They may certainly help you lose weight initially—only so that you regain it and end up being less healthy and more overweight. Such "die-ts" are for people who want something for nothing and who do not know much about how the body works. Your body literally dies on the diets. Let me give you a few examples.

High-carb and low-fat diets may help you in weight control, but only *some* of you, and specifically those of you who are endomorphs or those who digest food slowly. For others, such diets will increase fat due to increased insulin levels and loss of lean muscle tissue. Muscle is responsible for the basal metabolic rate (BMR), or the rate at which you burn calories of food at rest. High-carb and low-fat diets disturb your adrenal and thyroid functions (Wolcott, 307).

Such is also the case with high-protein and high-fat diets (e.g., Atkins' diet), which may help in weight control, but only for some body types (ectomorph predominant, or those who digest food fast). For others, such diets will increase fat because it lowers the BMR and creates a shortage of glucose. Whenever there is a shortage of glucose in the body, the body will break down its own muscle tissue for want of fuel. This is a vicious cycle since less muscle means lower metabolism and decreased ability to burn calories of fat. High-protein and high-fat diets cause mental fatigue and impair performance in your daily activities, and interfere with intense training (Wolcott, 307).

Protein-restricted diets are also not very good for most people, especially for individuals with an ectomorph body type or a mixed body type (ectomorph with mesomorph). Science has demonstrated that 98 percent of the cells in your body get replaced every year. For example, your body creates a new bone structure every 3 months. Every 6 weeks, all the cells in the liver get replaced. Every month you produce new skin. When you work out, you break down muscle (which is pure protein) and synthesize new lean tissue. In other words, every cell in the body gets continuously recycled (2 Hatfield, 530).

If you work out and consume inadequate amounts of protein, you will experience general fatigue, soreness, and you will not recover in time for your next workout. Even if a single amino acid (a building block of protein) is missing or low in the body, the synthesis of protein is stopped. Your whole training cycle will be thrown off because of your low recovery rate.

Balanced diets such as the zone diet 40-30-30 (carb/protein/fat) will also not work for everybody. It may work for mesomorphs, but for endomorphs and ectomorphs, it will increase fat. In the case of carb types (endomorphs), because it creates a shortage of glucose, the zone diet will make the body cannibalize its own muscle and, thus, lower the BMR. In the case of ectomorphs, due to an inadequate amount of protein, such a diet will decrease their lean body mass, thus lowering BMR (Wolcott, 307).

Chapter V
Physical Assessments

A few years ago, I came up with an accelerated program for my trainees and here is how it works. First of all, you fill out a Personal Achievement Goal Sheet. Naturally, it is based on your individual level of fitness, and the starting point will be different for all of us. It is up to your trainer and/or yourself, if you know how, to objectively assess your strengths and weaknesses and try to improve both. The goal sheet covers strength, cardio, nutrition, and other goals that are important facets of fitness. Fitness is not a fixed state but a continuum of many factors in your body and mind. That is why it is also crucial that you update your goals every month.

YOUR PERSONAL ACHIEVEMENT GOAL SHEET FOR THE MONTH OF ...

I. Strength training
   I will exercise _____ times a week, _____ minutes.

II. Cardiovascular training
   I will run _____ times a week, _____ minutes, target heart rate _____.

III. Proper nutrition and supplementation
   I will consume at least _____ meals a day, at least _____ calories total, take the following supplements daily _____, and make sure I eat from the following food categories:
   I will avoid/reduce/eliminate the following foods/additives:

IV. Lifestyle habits
   I will get at least _____ hours of sleep and make sure I spend some time daily on the activities I enjoy like _____.
   This is just a sample. You may, of course, come up with your own similar personal goal sheet that reflects other aspects of fitness.
   And here are some rules of the accelerated program:

TRANSCENDENTAL WARRIOR ACHIEVEMENT PROGRAM (TWAP)
PRINCIPLES, RULES, AND REGULATIONS

PRINCIPLES/GOALS

The TWAP program was designed to help you break through any barriers you have so far encountered on your way to complete fitness. TWAP works based on the principle of positive and negative reinforcement, which means that every month, you either win a prize or win a punishment workout.

To win a prize:
You must follow the PAG on a daily basis.

To win a punishment:
You fail to follow the PAG on a daily basis.

Rules:
Report to your trainer (or a workout buddy or a family member who supports you in your quest for fitness) every time you train with a green, yellow, or red card.

A green card means you followed each and every one of your monthly goals (see PAG).

A yellow card means you followed all but one of your monthly goals.

A red card means you did not follow at least two of your monthly goals.

Three yellow cards equal one red card. Each card summarizes your fitness activities from the time of your last workout till today's workout.

If you are on vacation or absolutely cannot make it to the gym and follow your monthly fitness activities, you cannot participate in TWAP for that month. If, having started the TWAP, you had to stop your fitness activities at the gym and you did not plan for it, your accumulated green cards can be used in the months to come. To win a monthly prize, you must not accumulate any red cards. You are allowed two yellow cards, however.

To win a punishment workout, you must accumulate at least one red card. Severity of your punishment workout will vary depending on the red cards you accumulated in that month.

If you forgot to bring your card to the workout session, you will automatically get a red card from your trainer unless you bring the card later that same day.

Aside from that, you can create your own Personal Record Sheet for specific physical attainments. Here is how mine looks. Of course, over the years, it will change as you improve and set new goals for yourself.

ANAEROBIC STRENGTH

Beginner's Krishna Warrior Fitness Challenge (BKWFC) workout time completion (warm-up not included): 28 minutes, 29 seconds

Calories burned without warm-up: 501

Maximum Heart Rate (MHR): 172 beats/minute

Average Heart Rate (AHR): 153 beats/minute

Loading parameters:

Sahadeva's Rocking Chair: 10 pounds held in both hands and feet

Hip-ups: 45-pound plate

Monster Jump: 25-pound plate

Walk-over Push-ups: 3 risers

Yudhisthira's Row: 130 pounds

Rakshasa Squats: 10 pounds held in each hand

Bhima's Running Wild Row: 120 pounds

IKWFC workout time completion (warm-up not included):

37 minutes, 16 seconds

Calories burned without warm-up: 620

MHR: 172 beats/minute

AHR: 148 beats/minute

Loading parameters:

Nakula's J Cross: 10 pounds each arm

Krishna Warrior Curl: 35 pounds, 15 pounds on stretched out arm

Karna's Fall: 25-pound plate

Low Cable Uppercuts: 35 pounds each arm

Kung Fu Triceps Ext: 25 pounds

Asvatthama's Row: 80 pounds

Flying Eagle: 10 pounds each arm

Eccentric Sit-up: 25-pound plate

AKWFC workout time completion: 38 minutes, 29 seconds

Calories burned without warm-up: 701

MHR: 181 beats/minute

AHR: 162 beats/minute

Loading parameters:

Core Master: 50 pounds

Small Kangaroo Jumps: 45-pound plate

Explosive Push-ups: 3 risers

ABSOLUTE STRENGTH

Bench-press with dumbbells without assistance:
200 pounds/9 consecutive repetitions/without assistance, lowering dumbbells to 90-degree angle
Military dumbbell press without assistance:
140 pounds (two 70-pound dumbbells)
6 consecutive repetitions

Olympic Squat without assistance:
385 pounds/8 consecutive repetitions/without assistance, bending legs to approximately a 90-degree angle
One-legged Squat with 60 pounds (two 30-pound dumbbells)
6 consecutive repetitions/3 sets/going all the way down until butt touches heel. Both legs.

Specific Absolute Strength:

One-armed, One-foot Push-ups:
Right arm: 10 consecutive repetitions/4 sets/going at least halfway down or lower without putting down the foot that's supposed to be in the air.
Left arm: 8 consecutive repetitions
One-armed, two-finger push-ups
5 consecutive repetitions each arm

Specific Strength Endurance:
One-armed push-ups
30 consecutive repetitions going at least halfway down with shoulders and hips aligned. Exercise both arms.

Anaerobic Linear Strength Endurance:
Push-ups
1,000 repetitions in 30 minutes
200 consecutive push-ups
Medium-grip chin-ups
30 consecutive repetitions
1 mile run: 5 minutes, 21 seconds

Aerobic Linear Strength Endurance:
Marathon run 3 hours, 19 minutes, 32 seconds

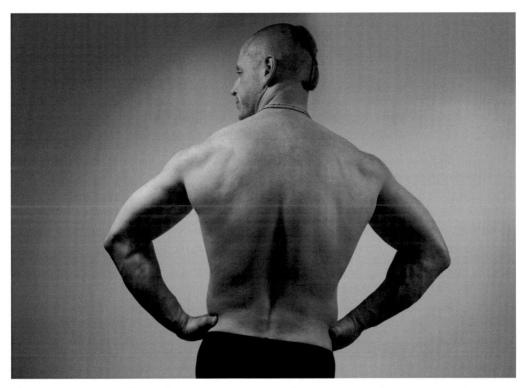

If you were not able to break a new record today or perform at your best, do not be discouraged. There is always tomorrow. Remember, it is about your mind-set. So set the mind on Krishna, because it all depends on Him!

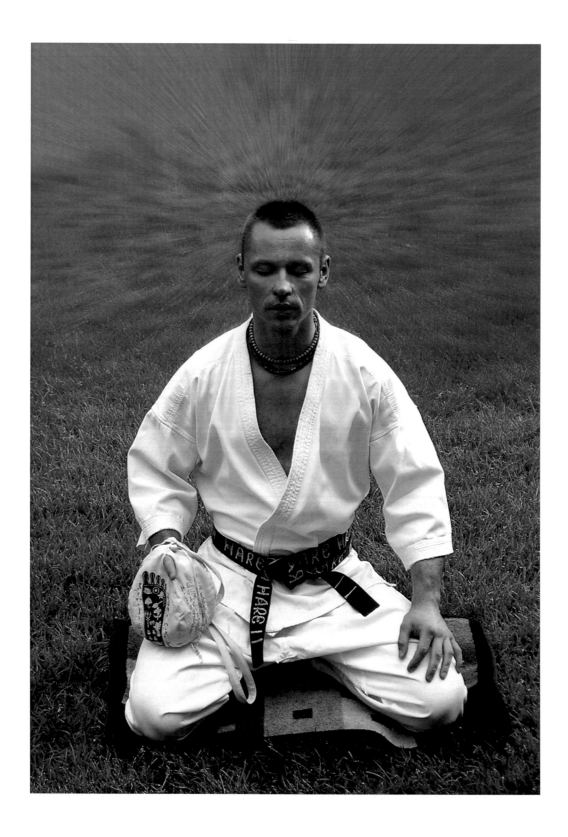

Chapter VI

Spiritual Technologies of a Krishna Warrior

Spiritual factors are part of health, fitness, and, therefore, physical performance at all levels. A three-time world champion in power lifting and the founder of the International Sports Sciences Association (ISSA), Dr. Frederick Hatfield is clear on the matter of spiritual factors when he explains (1 Hatfield 85) his strength theory. "Spiritual factors: Without becoming embroiled in a philosophical discussion regarding the merits of one religion or another, my strong belief is that if you are spiritually at peace with your Creator, all things are possible. If you don't believe in and practice this in your everyday life, then how can your life—and your quest for fitness—even have meaning?"

CHARACTER QUALITIES OF KRISHNA WARRIORS

One of the greatest assets of a Krishna warrior is his ability to focus and evoke the power divine. We are not just talking about the power to focus and break an ice block or bench press 500 pounds. As you will soon learn, physical strength is a kind of power. But Krishna warriors are all about the power to channel the positive spiritual energy to another person by accessing the energy of the Supreme Warrior, or God. The Lord's fighters are always assured of protection, victory, and happiness in his eternal service. What follows is a list of character qualities and, later, a list of rare benefits acquired by those who fully engage in Krishna Warrior Fitness Challenge practice with faith and determination.

"The Supreme Personality of Godhead said: Fearlessness; purification of one's existence; cultivation of spiritual knowledge; charity; self-control; performance of sacrifice; study of the scriptures; austerity; simplicity; nonviolence; truthfulness; freedom from anger; renunciation; tranquility; aversion to faultfinding; compassion for all living entities; freedom from covetousness; gentleness; modesty; steady determination; vigor; forgiveness; fortitude; cleanliness; and freedom from envy and from the passion for honor—these transcendental qualities belong to godly men endowed with divine nature" (1 Prabhupada 740).

Krishna further explains the characteristics of those who have transcended the mental and intellectual levels of existence by serving the Lord. "He who does not hate illumination, attachment, and delusion when they are present or long for them when they disappear; who is unwavering and undisturbed through all these reactions of the material qualities, remaining neutral and transcendental, knowing that the material nature alone is active; who is situated in the self and regards alike happiness and distress; who looks upon a lump of earth, a stone, and a piece of gold with an equal eye; who is equal toward the desirable and the undesirable; who is steady, situated equally well in praise and blame, honor and dishonor; who treats alike both friend and enemy; and who has renounced all material activities—such a person is said to have transcended the material nature" (1 Prabhupada 704).

RARE BENEFITS KRISHNA WARRIORS RECEIVE (6 PRABHUPADA 3)

1. Immediate relief from all kinds of material distress.
2. All-auspiciousness.
3. Enjoyment of spiritual pleasure.
4. The ability to attract the protection and love of the Supreme Warrior, Krishna.

It is important that we understand these benefits. In the material world, the spiritual body is dormant and the material body manifest. The purpose of exercising your body, mind, and spirit is to restore ourselves to our constitutional nature: to manifest the dormant spiritual body and dissolve the body made of material elements. Although a Krishna warrior will remain connected externally with the material (gross and subtle) body until death, he will have already rediscovered his actual identity as the Supreme Lord's servant. This is why he will always be protected by the Supreme Warrior and enjoy pleasure on the spiritual platform of the soul. Such pleasure transcends gross or subtle sense enjoyment (for more information on this matter, read my *Transcendental Warrior* trilogy). Happiness on the spiritual platform is ever-increasing, eternal, and without bounds.

Simply by fully engaging in the Krishna Warrior Fitness Challenge—even before completely conquering our weakness—we can begin to experience both relief from material distress and spiritual pleasure in our work. Even when we undergo the same material tribulations such as sickness or injury, we will not become disturbed, because we know who we are and what our purpose is. This knowledge is on a completely different platform than how we have previously thought of ourselves. It is knowledge of the soul.

Once we conquer the mind, the covered divine qualities will shine forth like those of other great spiritual warriors. Those qualities will destroy all material qualities imposed upon us by our obstinate mind. Srimad-Bhagavatam (3 Prabhupada 638) confirms: "One who attains pure unalloyed devotional service to the Supreme Lord develops all the good qualities of the demigods, whereas a person who does not develop such service, despite all material qualifications, is sure to go astray, for he hovers on the mental platform."

Even in the beginning of the fight, good qualities begin to manifest in us. We will, thus, become all-auspicious, capable of emanating a spiritual influence over others, inspiring them to also begin a life dedicated to God. Therefore, we will attract and benefit everyone, since all living entities unknowingly desire the same spiritual nature that is now temporarily covered by material energy. These results can never be obtained by belonging to organizations based on something other than essential spirituality.

Pure qualities are found only in the soul, never in the conditioned, material body or mind. Those who endeavor to develop patience, tolerance, forgiveness, and nonviolence without the correct motive will find themselves further entangled in matter. The purpose of developing the types of qualities listed below is simply to facilitate our service to the Supreme Warrior and to truly help people. These qualities lie dormant in the heart of every living entity because each living entity is essentially a servant of the Supreme Lord. Only by awakening this realization can those original qualities be called forth in their spiritual form.

Now here is the sound vibration that descends from the spiritual world and is the spiritual technology on which Krishna Warriors rely in their quest for holistic fitness. This vibration, or mantra, will allow all warriors to transcend all mental and physical difficulties and, thus, become fully determined on their life mission, whatever that mission may mean to each of them personally.

CHANTING FOR ALL TIMES

There are countless verses in the books of knowledge that recommend chanting of the Supreme Lord's holy name as the only means of reaching perfect consciousness. Chanting is loving service offered to the Lord. Here are some of these verses.

While on the battlefield of Kurukshetra, the Lord enlightens the warrior Arjuna with these words: "Always chanting My glories, endeavoring with great determination, bowing down before Me, these great souls perpetually worship Me with devotion" (1 Prabhupada 474).

In the New Testament, St. Paul echoes that "whoever calls upon the name of the Lord will be saved" (Romans 10.13). In the Old Testament, the Psalms encourage us to praise the Lord's name from the rising of the sun to its setting. "Your name, O God, like your praise, reaches the ends of the earth" (48.10). "I will lift up my hands and call on your name. My soul is satisfied and my mouth praises you with joyful lips when I think of you on my bed and mediate on you in the watches of the night" (63.4–6). "Make a joyful noise to God, all the earth; sing the glory of his name" (66.1–2). "I will sing of your might; I will sing aloud of your steadfast love in the morning. . . . I will sing praises to you, for you, O God, are my fortress . . ." (59.16–17).

Lord Krishna assures us that He is no different than the sound vibration of Hare Krishna. In the Sri Chaitanya-Caritamrita (2 Prabhupada 708), it is stated: "In this fallen age of Iron, the holy name of the Lord, the Hare Krishna *maha-mantra*, is the incarnation of Lord Krishna. Simply by chanting the holy name, one associates with the Lord directly. Anyone who does this is certainly delivered."

Master Prabhupada[30] explains (1 Prabhupada 427) that Krishna's holy name contains the sacred syllable "om." Om contains the impersonal aspect of the Absolute Truth, or Brahman, whereas, the sound vibration "Krishna" contains all three aspects of the Absolute Truth, namely the God in the heart (Supersoul), the impersonal energy of God, and God Himself.

THE SUBLIME POWER OF THE HARE KRISHNA SOUND VIBRATION

Now hear Master Orayen's explanation of the secret potency of the sound vibration that will empower you to carry out your mission and become victorious.

The transcendental vibration established by the chanting of *Hare Krishna, Hare Krishna, Krishna Krishna, Hare, Hare, Hare Rama, Hare Rama, Rama, Rama, Hare, Hare,* is the sublime method for reviving our transcendental consciousness. As living, spiritual souls, we are all originally Krishna-conscious entities, but due to our association with matter from time immemorial, our consciousness is now adulterated by the material atmosphere. The material atmosphere, in which we are now living, is called *maya,* or illusion. *Maya* means "that which is not."

And what is this illusion? The illusion is that we are all trying to be lords of material nature, while actually we are under the grip of her stringent laws. When a servant artificially tries to imitate the all-powerful master, it is called illusion. We are trying to exploit the resources of material nature, but actually, we are becoming more and more entangled in her complexities.

Therefore, although we are engaged in a hard struggle to conquer nature, we are ever more dependent on her. This illusory struggle against material nature can be stopped at once by revival of our eternal Krishna consciousness.

Hare Krishna, Hare Krishna, Krishna Krishna, Hare, Hare is the transcendental process for reviving this original, pure consciousness. By chanting this transcendental vibration, we can cleanse away all misgivings within our hearts. The basic principle of all such misgivings is the false consciousness that "I am the lord of all I survey."

Krishna consciousness is not an artificial imposition on the mind. This consciousness is the original natural energy of the living entity. When we hear the transcendental vibration, this consciousness is revived. This simplest method of meditation is recommended for this age.

By practical experience, one can perceive that by chanting this *maha-mantra,* or the Great Chanting for Deliverance, one can at once feel a transcendental ecstasy coming through from the spiritual stratum. In the material concept of life, we are busy in the matter of sense gratification, as if we were in the lower animal stage. A little elevated from this status of sense gratification, one is engaged in mental speculation for the purpose of getting out of the material clutches. A little elevated from this speculative status, when one is intelligent enough, one tries to find out the supreme cause of all causes—within and without. And when one is factually on the plane of spiritual understanding, surpassing the stages of sense, mind, and intelligence, he is then on the transcendental plane. This chanting of the Hare Krishna mantra is enacted from the spiritual platform, and, thus, this sound vibration surpasses all lower strata of consciousness—namely sensual, mental, and intellectual.

There is no need, therefore, to understand the language of the mantra, nor is there any need for mental speculation nor any intellectual adjustment for chanting this *maha-mantra.* It is automatic, from the spiritual platform, and as such, anyone can take part in vibrating this transcendental sound without any previous qualification. In a more advanced stage, of course, one is not expected to commit offenses on grounds of spiritual understanding.

In the beginning, there may not be the presence of all transcendental ecstasies, which are eight in number. These are: (1) being stopped as though dumb, (2) perspiration, (3) standing up of hairs on the body, (4) dislocation of voice, (5) trembling, (6) fading of the body, (7) crying in ecstasy, and (8) trance.

There is no doubt that chanting for a while takes one immediately to the spiritual platform, and one shows the first symptom of this in the urge to dance along with the chanting of the mantra. We have seen this. Even a child can take part in the chanting and dancing.

Of course, for one who is too entangled in material life, it takes a little more time to come to this point, but even such a materially engrossed man is raised to the spiritual platform very quickly. When it is chanted by a pure devotee of the Lord in love, it has the greatest efficacy on hearers, and as such, this chanting should be heard from the lips of a pure devotee of the Lord, so that immediate effects can be achieved. As far as possible, chanting from the lips of nondevotees should be avoided. Milk touched by the lips of a serpent has poisonous effects.

The word *Hara* is the form of addressing the energy of the Lord, and the words *Krishna* and *Rama* are forms of addressing the Lord himself. Both Krishna and Rama mean the supreme pleasure, and Hara is the supreme pleasure energy of the Lord, changed to Hare (Haray) in the vocative. The supreme pleasure energy of the Lord helps us to reach the Lord.

The material energy, called *maya*, is also one of the multienergies of the Lord. And we the living entities are also the energy, marginal energy, of the Lord. The living entities are described as superior to material energy. When the superior energy is in contact with the inferior energy, an incompatible situation arises, but when the superior marginal energy is in contact with the superior energy, called Hara, it is established in its happy, normal condition.

These three words, namely *Hara*, *Krishna*, and *Rama*, are the transcendental seeds of the *maha-mantra*. The chanting is a spiritual call for the Lord and his energy, to give protection to the conditioned soul. This chanting is exactly like the genuine cry of a child for its mother's presence. Mother Hara helps the devotee achieve the Lord Father's grace, and the Lord reveals himself to the devotee who chants this mantra sincerely.

No other means of spiritual realization is as effective in this age of quarrel and hypocrisy as the *maha-mantra: Hare Krishna, Hare Krishna, Krishna, Krishna, Hare, Hare, Hare Rama, Hare Rama, Rama, Rama, Hare Hare* (7 Prabhupada p. 146).

THE 10 OFFENSES AGAINST THE HOLY NAME
(BASED ON 6 PRABHUPADA 72)

As with any authorized medicinal preparation, to receive the full benefit of chanting Hare Krishna, one must take precautions not to misuse it:

1. Do not blaspheme devotees who have dedicated their lives to spreading the glories of the Lord's holy name. No Krishna warrior, whether neophyte or champion, should be blasphemed. All warriors are dear to the Lord, and he will not tolerate their being reviled. Those who do so will lose their power and will find themselves unable to utilize either their weapons or the potion of the holy name.

2. Warriors should not consider the names of the demigods, such as Lord Brahma and Lord Shiva, to be equal to or independent of, the name of Lord Vishnu.[31]

3. Warriors should not disobey or minimize the orders of their spiritual masters.

4. Warriors should not blaspheme Vedic (spiritual scriptures from India) literature or literature in pursuance of the Vedic version. This includes books of knowledge written by strict adherents to the spiritual path who may refer to other authorized scriptures and masters while writing their unique realizations. Such books are considered as good as the original Vedas. They are written to address spiritual issues according to timely concerns.

5. Warriors should not consider the glories of chanting Hare Krishna as imagination.

6. Warriors should not give some mundane interpretation on the Lord's holy name.

7. Warriors should not commit sins on the strength of chanting the Lord's holy name. The holy name is not meant for atonement but for glorification of the Lord.

8. A warrior should not consider the chanting of the holy name to be one of the ritualistic activities offered in the Vedas as materially motivated activities. Such activities, as Krishna tells Arjuna, are detrimental to the attainment of spiritual consciousness: "Men of small knowledge are very much attached to the flowery words of the Vedas, which recommend various fruitive [material, result-oriented] activities for elevation to heavenly planets, resultant good birth, power, and so forth. . . . In the minds of those who are too attached to sense enjoyment and material opulence, and who are bewildered by such things, the resolute determination for devotional service to the Supreme Lord does not take place" (Bhagavad-Gita As It Is 2.42–44).

9. Warriors should not instruct faithless persons in the intimate glories of the holy name. We should spread the science of chanting the holy name of God in the war against materialistic consciousness, but we should not deliver more confidential knowledge about the holy name's identity to those who are not ready to hear it. It is sufficient to present the benefits of chanting as loving service to Lord Krishna, but not necessary to explain more intimate understandings of the holy name to those who are not qualified by faith. Otherwise, those who are still bound by matter may commit offenses against the holy name, and our teaching will have been a kind of violence toward them.

10. A warrior should have complete faith in the chanting of the holy name and not maintain material attachments after having understood so many instructions on this matter.

If we are attentive while we are chanting, we will find the strength to realize the power of Krishna, whereas inattentive chanting will remain mechanical and will not be strengthening. Chanting means reciting the Lord's name. It is a kind of invitation to the Lord to receive our worship and respect. If we remain inattentive even as we invite the Lord, then we are acting offensively and will not find ourselves empowered.

HOW TO CHANT THE HOLY NAME
(BASED ON VIKASA 28–31):

Here are some simple directions about how to drink the nectar of the holy name:

1. Obtain your beads from an authorized temple of International Society for Krishna Consciousness (ISKCON). You should also get a bead bag to protect your beads. The bag is useful, because it enables you to take your beads anywhere. You can chant anywhere and at any time, and, thus, enhance your spiritual consciousness by evoking more of the Lord's mercy.

2. Once you have your beads, hold them in your right hand. Offer thanks and respects to Master Orayen for the gift of the Holy Name he has kindly given you.

3. On your string of beads, you will find a head bead. You will recognize it because it is larger than the others and usually has a tassel or loop coming from it. Grasp the first bead on one side of the head bead (doesn't matter which side) between your right thumb and middle finger. Your index finger should not touch the bead.

4. Roll the bead back and forth between your thumb and middle finger (to engage the sense of touch) and chant *Hare Krishna, Hare Krishna, Krishna, Krishna, Hare, Hare, Hare Rama, Hare Rama, Rama, Rama, Hare, Hare.* (*Hare* is pronounced "Ha-ray." *Rama* rhymes with "drama.") Say each syllable of each word as clearly as you can. Concentrate on the sound of each word.

5. When you have chanted all 16 divine words once, move your thumb and middle finger to the next bead and chant the mantra again.

6. In this way, chant on all 108 beads until you have again come to the head bead. Do not chant on the head bead. You have completed one round, or one mouthful of nectar. Offer your respects and thanks to Master Prabhupada again.

7. Before proceeding to the second round, turn your set of beads around in your hand and chant in the other direction. Do not cross the head bead to continue chanting. Then chant your second round. Similarly, you can chant 16 rounds.

Always treat your beads with respect. Don't let them touch the floor, your feet, anything unclean, or take them into the bathroom.[32]

If you are unable to commit to chanting a full 16 rounds, know that even one round of the mantra will give you strength and help you progress. Gradually, try to raise to the standard. But you should realize that the amount of spiritual power available to you will only increase as you drink the right amount. As in any martial science, you have to practice as your master instructs, and 16 rounds is the standard set by Master Prabhupada for warriors from the West. When you follow his instructions, he will bless you with realization and ability.

Arsenal Three

And More Training

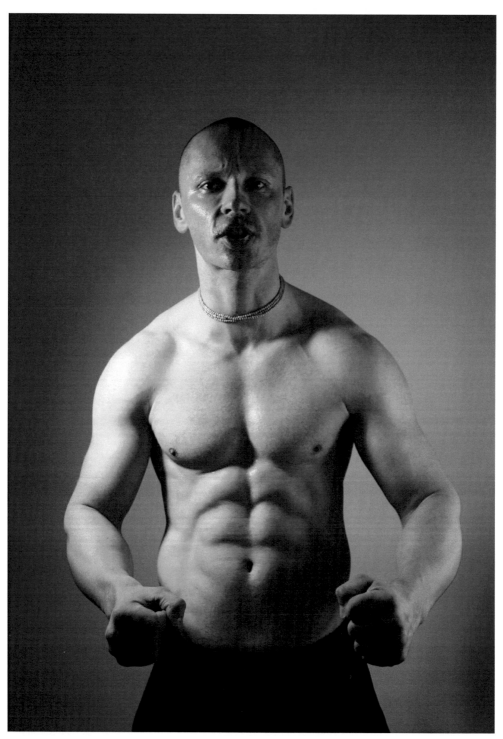

Do not enter here unless you have passed through the three levels!

Chapter VII

Exercise Treasury Chest

Since you have proven yourselves to be dedicated to your warrior PATH, I will treat you with more exercises. They are divided into Upper, Core Upper, Core, Core Lower, and Combination segments.

What you can do is arrange them appropriately to create new Peripheral Heart Action routines as demonstrated in the three mesocycles you have completed. For example, to create a single sequence of a three-level PHA workout, I would choose Hanuman Monkey Pull, Dynamic Crunch, and Karate Punch.

Try to build sequences in such a way that each exercise's main muscle (prime mover) is away from the main muscle of the exercise that follows. This reinforces the cardio effect. For example, Hanuman Monkey Pull utilizes biceps brachii as the prime mover, Dynamic Crunch works abdominals and obliques (sides), and Karate Punch utilizes rear shoulders as prime movers (it also pumps a lot of blood into your gluteus maximus, which is part of your lower body, and that's another reason I picked it as the last exercise). So there is a considerable amount of blood going from arms to core and back to arms.

A good PHA loop involves one exercise for upper body, one for core, and one for lower body (prime movers considered). Feel free to add your own exercises to the treasury or even to the Krishna Warrior Fitness Challenge program and modify sequences while adhering to this PHA principle.

UPPER

Hanuman Monkey Pull

Jumping Crocodiles

Abhimanyu's Karate Pump

CORE AND UPPER BODY

Core Master (CM) Rear Shoulder Circle

Ark's Fly

CM Dumbbell Shoulder Raise

Ab Master (AM) Alternated Dumbbell Raise

Ghatotkacha's Curl

AM Alternated Shoulder Circles

Bhima's Core Hold

CORE

Dynamic Crunch

Isometric Side Crunch

Arjuna's Rocking Side Crunch

Hanuman's Circles

Dhrstaketu's Jackknives

CORE AND LOWER BODY

Circle Kick on Vertical Abdominal Bench

Reverse Circle Vertical Abdominal Bench

Roman Ts

COMBINATIONS

Balarama's Circles

Bhima's Shoulder Rover

Garuda Shoulder Lift

Karate Punch

Upper (mainly arms involved as prime movers and doing most of the work)

Hanuman Monkey Pull/Hanging From Bar Single Biceps Pull

Difficulty level: I

Caution: If you have shoulder problems, you may be able to perform the exercise modification provided.

Origin: ID

Presenter: Warrior Susan

Starting position:

Here, you can easily use the well-known Smith's Machine (normally used for squatting, bench pressing). Lift the bar and set it at your eye level. Stand 2 feet away from the bar with your left shoulder toward it. Grasp the bar with your left hand using a palm-down grip. Place your right foot in front of the left foot so that the heel of the right foot touches the toes of the left one. Raise your right arm so it is aligned with the left shoulder. Look straight ahead (see Photo 7.1).

Movement:

While holding the bar with your left hand, slowly pull yourself up to the left and then away from the bar by letting your left arm extend through its full range (see Photos 7.2–7.3). Make sure your torso and hips remain aligned during the execution of this movement and all the muscles are kept tight (especially in the lower and midback) so the body moves as one unit. You should stay as rigid as an iron stick, and the only movement that moves the whole body occurs at the elbow joint. Once you extend yourself fully to the right, immediately contract your biceps again and pull yourself back up the same way you came before. Do it 15 times on each arm.

Major muscles involved:

The prime mover in the Hanuman Pull is the front of your arm, or biceps brachii. The assisting muscle is upper and middle trapezius (upper back). Torso-stabilizing muscles are erector spinae (lower back)

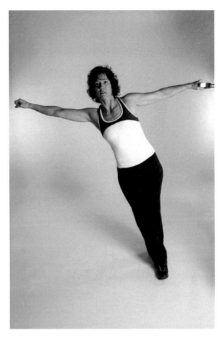

Photo 7.1

and external oblique. The main muscle being used in the free hand that remains extended in the air is medial deltoid (shoulder).

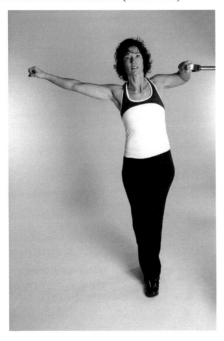

Photo 7.2

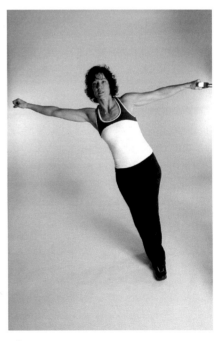

Photo 7.3

Ark's tips:
Perform this exercise slowly and pull through your shoulder. Do not deviate from the vertical plane, which runs through the body from front to back (it divides it into left and right portions). If you feel this exercise is not stressing your biceps or upper back sufficiently, you probably need to reposition the feet. Bring them closer to the bar for a better extension of the arm. You can also hold a light dumbbell or plate in your free hand to target the medial deltoid (shoulder) there.

Breathing technique:
Inhale as you move away from the bar and exhale as you approach the bar.

Sports applications:
The Hanuman Pull will help swimmers due to its tremendous stress on the upper back muscle. It will also help in sports that require great gripping strength, such as rock climbing, judo (throwing), archery (stringing the bow), and others.

Modification exercise (for persons with shoulder conditions):
Perform a simple pull-down on a machine or cable pull-down station. Use a narrow undergrip.

Jumping Crocodiles/Explosive Forward Jumps on Two Knuckles

Difficulty Level: S

Caution: If you have shoulder problems or weak wrists, you may be able to perform the exercise modification provided.

Origin: K

Presenter: Warrior Greg

Starting position:
Position yourself on a mat in a push-up position on your knuckles rather than open palms. Make sure that you are using the first two knuckles as they are the strongest of the five. Specifically put more emphasis on the first knuckle (about 70 percent). Also, make sure that your hand is in a neutral position and the elbows are close to your body. Go down in a push-up so your chin is almost touching the floor. See Photo 7.4.

Movement:
Look straight ahead and keep your chin up. Tighten up all the muscles, especially your hands and arms. Using all of the body's muscles, propel yourself up and forward so both the hands and feet come off the floor for a split second. Land and immediately explode again. See Photos 7.5–7.10.

Major muscles involved:
There are many muscles at work here. Clavicular pectoralis muscles (upper chest) are involved, although you may not really feel them a lot. Triceps brachii (back of arm) is the prime mover for this exercise. It is doing a tremendous amount of work at the pushing-up

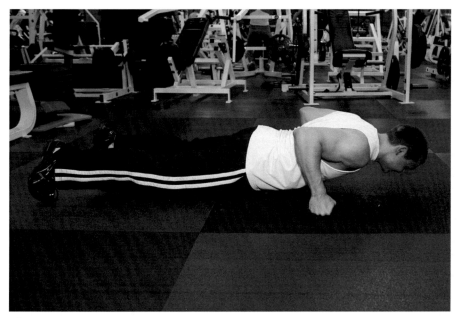

Photo 7.4

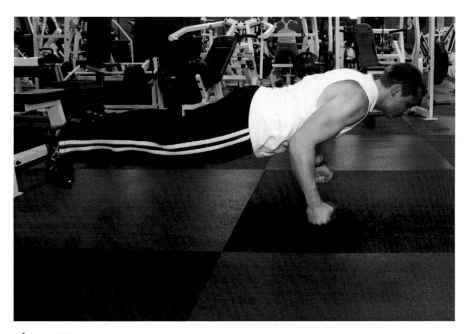

Photo 7.5

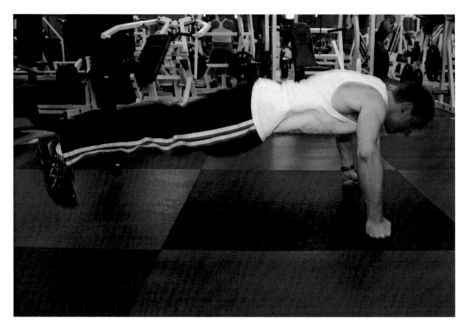

Photo 7.6

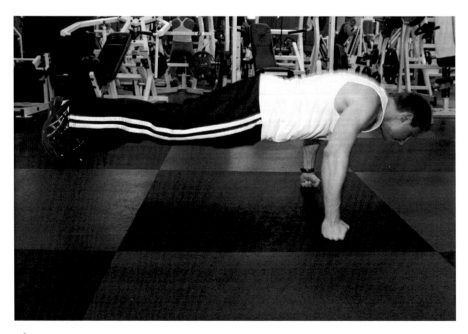

Photo 7.7

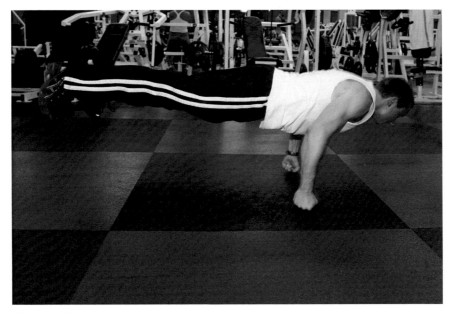

Photo 7.8

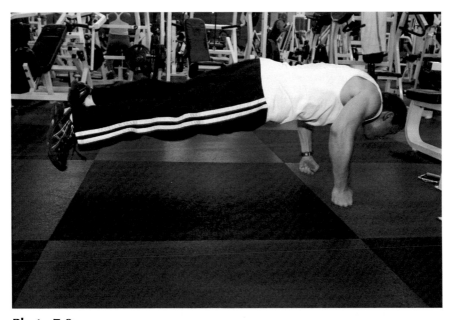

Photo 7.9

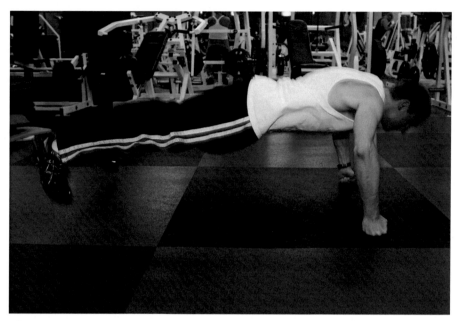

Photo 7.10

motion and landing. Anterior deltoid (front shoulder) muscle is assisting the pectoralis and triceps brachii muscles in the pushing motion. The pushing-up motion forces the rectus abdominis as well as external oblique muscles (sides) to stabilize your core to facilitate jumping and landing. Another stabilizing muscle in the Jumping Crocodile is latissimus dorsi (side of back). Serratus anterior is also part of the stabilizing muscle group.

Ark's tips:
You better keep those fists and wrists tight unless you want to break them! It is best you practice simple push-ups on these two knuckles before you attempt this feat. This exercise is for the superstrong, and superstrong does not mean that you can bench or squat a lot. It is functional superstrength. Do you want to try it backwards too?

Breathing technique:
Exhale as you take off and inhale as you land. Breathing is very forceful and fast in this exercise.

Sports applications:
There are few exercises as effective in developing punching power as Jumping Crocodiles. Most martial artists can derive great benefits from it. Because the exercise is executed on the knuckles that you punch with, it will toughen them up. Jumping Crocodiles also will prepare a martial artist to receive a blow to the torso (stomach, ribs, shoulder) by maximally tensing up those muscles for split seconds.

More than anything, a martial artist will improve the starting strength of his/her punch as well as its descend phase (eccentric strength). Sport disciplines that will benefit from Jumping Crocodiles are football (pushing) and gymnastics (free exercises), among others.

Modification exercise (for persons with shoulder conditions or weak wrists):
Perform regular push-ups. Make sure not to bend your arms more than 90 degrees.

Abhimanyu's Karate Pump/One-armed Narrow Push-up on Two Knuckles

Difficulty Level: S

Caution: If you have shoulder problems or weak wrists, you may be able to perform the exercise modification provided.

Origin: IDP

Presenter: Warrior Greg

Starting position:
Position yourself on a mat in a push-up position on your knuckles rather than open palms. Make sure that you are using the first two knuckles as they are the strongest of the five. Specifically put more emphasis on the first knuckle (about 70 percent). Lift your right hand and place it behind your back (see Photo 7.11).

Movement:
Commence Abhimanyu's Karate Pump by bending your left arm until your biceps and forearm touch. Make sure to keep the elbow in rather than out. Maintain high muscle tension.

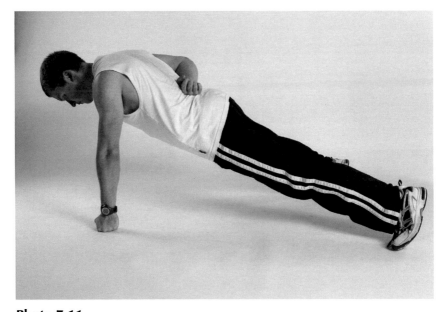

Photo 7.11

You are now in a low push-up position with hips and shoulders even. Without resting, push up and return to the original position. Stay in the five to eight repetition range for this exercise. See Photos 7.12–16. Switch arms.

Major muscles involved:

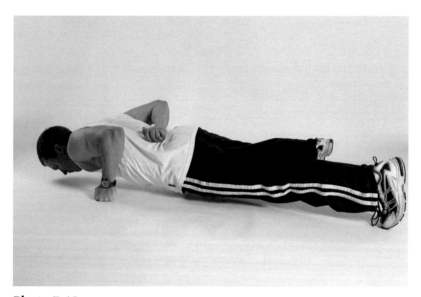

Photo 7.12

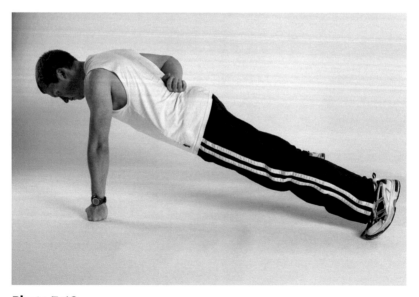

Photo 7.13

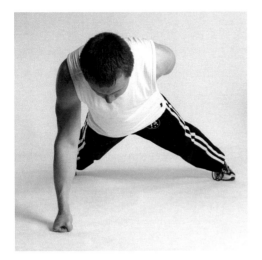 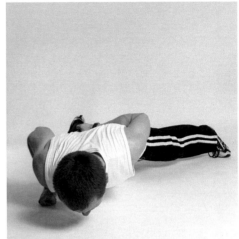

Photo 7.14   **Photo 7.15**

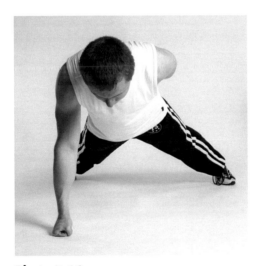

Photo 7.16

As this exercise is very specific to punching sports (karate, kickboxing, etc.), you will need to keep the elbow close to your side (almost touching it). In this way, you will involve the very same muscles in the same way as in a punch. Triceps brachii (back of arm) is the prime mover and clavicular pectoralis (upper chest) is the assisting mover in the exercise. Anterior deltoid (front shoulder) is assisting in the movement. Core muscles (abdominals, obliques), as well as the sides of the back (latissimus dorsi) are stabilizing the trunk to make the pushing motion possible.

Ark's tips:
Focus on maintaining high muscle tension, warrior! Go slow! Don't rush through this exercise and do it incorrectly. Make sure your abdominal wall is very hard before you go down and push back up. Keep yourself very tight, rock-solid, including the neck. You are not supposed to relax when you are very close to the floor. Do not compromise proper form. Keep those shoulders and hips even (aligned)!

Breathing technique:
Inhale as you go down and hold your breath as you push up. Once you get over the sticking point, powerfully exhale. Take a couple of quick breaths and go down again.

Sports application:
Here is a great exercise for developing maximum strength of one's punch. More than anything, you will improve your maximum strength by doing the Abhimanyu's Karate Pump. Maximum strength phase of training should come after you have sufficiently increased your muscle size. Other sport disciplines that will benefit from the triceps push-off are football (pushing), tennis (forehand), and gymnastics (free exercises).

Modification (for persons with shoulder conditions or weak wrists):
Perform regular push-ups but do not bend arms more than 90 degrees.

OK, I know you want to keep reading. So here you go. I am throwing in this ultimate progression to the Abhimanyu Pump.

Come on, warrior, you're not done yet!/progression:
Take one foot off the floor. In this case, it would be your left foot. Remember the great warrior Abhimanyu when you pump it up!

Core and Upper Body (most work is performed by prime moving upper muscles, but also a lot of core is used for stabilization)

CM Rear Shoulder Circle on Mat

Difficulty level: A

Caution: If you have back problems, you may be able to perform the exercise modification provided.

Origin: ID

Presenter: Self

Starting position:
Position yourself on a mat. Hold a light dumbbell in your left hand. Place your right hand on the mat next to your thigh. Supporting your body with your right hand, raise both legs straight up in the air to about 45 degrees from the floor. Lean back and arch. Keep the chin up. Your body should form the letter "V" when seen from the side (see Photo 7.17).

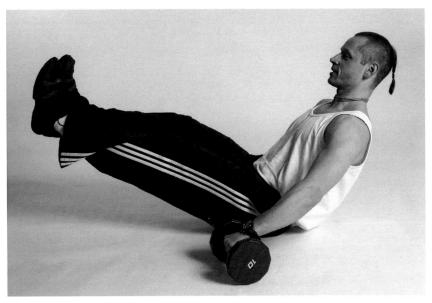

Photo 7.17

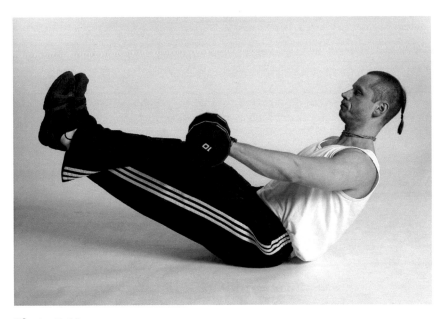

Photo 7.18

Movement:
Using a palm-down grip, raise the dumbbell slightly over your head and continue behind your head and to the side and down, making a full circle (see Photos 7.18–21). Medium tempo is appropriate for this exercise. Repeat 15 times and switch hands.

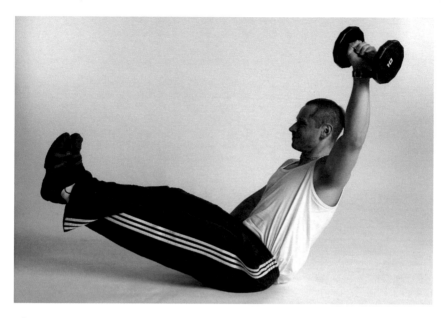

Photo 7.19

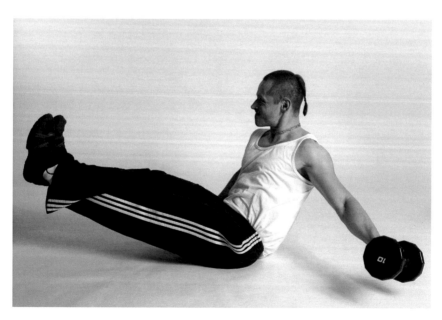

Photo 7.20

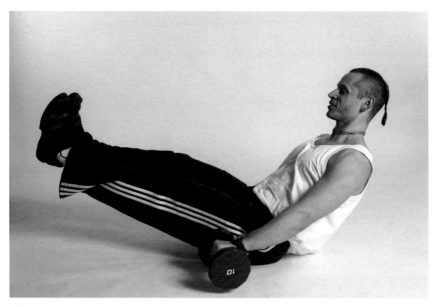

Photo 7.21

Major muscles involved:
There are quite a few of them at work here! First of all, by holding the "V" position, you work rectus femoris (upper front thigh), rectus abdominis (especially lower abdominals), and erector spinae (mid- and lower back). These are your stabilizing muscles, and they contract isometrically, or without lengthening and shortening. Second, in the arm, you work the anterior deltoid (front shoulder) and your posterior deltoid (rear shoulder). The front shoulder is the prime mover for the arm.

Ark's tips:
It is crucial to maintain the "V" shape. Otherwise, your back will round, and you will create unnecessary strain on the spinal cord.

Breathing technique:
Exhale upon raising the dumbbell and inhale when lowering it.

Sports applications:
Core Master Rear Circles force you to contract trunk muscles isometrically (without flexing or extending) in a suspended position. The essence of this exercise lies in working the core so athletes like gymnasts, dancers, martial artists, and football players alike, will derive great benefit from it. As far as the Shoulder Circle is concerned, we can again give the example of *karateka*. The *karateka* is required to keep hands up on guard at all times, which requires one to constantly maintain a state of isometric contraction in the muscles and execute powerful motions every few seconds. This calls for muscular endurance of fibers in the front shoulder

muscle. There are many sports like boxing, wrestling, or football (linemen who block or hit their opponents) that call for the raising of the arms on a consistent basis and, thus, the arm raise will improve endurance of those muscle fibers.

Modification (for extension-biased persons[33]):
Stand up and perform the same movement. You can also sit in a recline position and perform the movement. This way, your spine will get more support. Immediately after that, you can do a set of Crunches.

> Ark's Fly/Core Master (CM) Single Fly on Cables with Legs Up
>
> Difficulty level: A
>
> Caution: If you have back or shoulder problems, you may be able to perform the exercise modification provided.
>
> Origin: ID
>
> Presenter: Self

Starting position:
Position a flat bench between two cable stations. You should be able to adjust the height of each pulley to its lowest notch on the cable station. Next, attach two handles to each one of the cables. Adjust the weight as desired. Holding one handle of the cable, sit somewhere in the middle of the bench. The cables can be aligned with your shoulders (but it is not required). Next, with one hand, tightly grab the edge of the bench you are sitting on and try to balance yourself on your tailbone by lifting up your two legs and entire torso (see Photo 7.22). Your body should form the letter "V" when side-viewed (see Photo 7.23). Hold your legs straight in the knees and keep your chest forward, back arched.

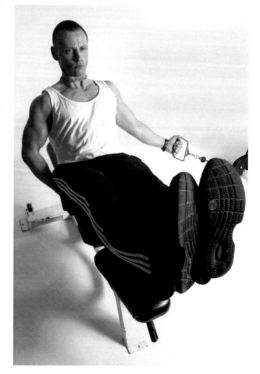

Movement:
Slowly extend the arm that's holding the handle of the cable down and to the side. The arm should be slightly bent. While holding the letter "V," position pull your arm up against the resistance created by the pulley (see Photos 7.24–26). Then slowly return to the starting position. Perform at least 12 repetitions. Switch arms.

Photo 7.22

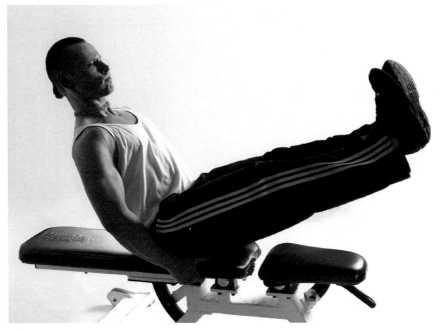

Photo 7.23

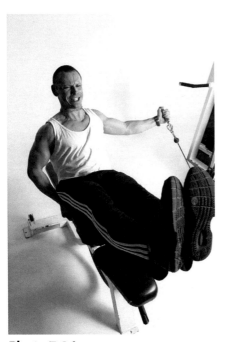

Photo 7.24

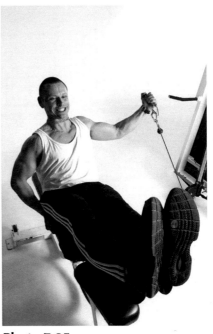

Photo 7.25

Major muscles involved:
There are quite a variety of muscles involved here. First of all, by holding the position correctly, you isometrically involve rectus abdominis (especially the lower portion), transverse abdominis, erector spinae, and rectus femoris (upper thighs). When performing the Fly concentrically, you work clavicular pectoralis major and/or sternal pectoralis major (depending on how much the pulley is aligned with your shoulders). In the eccentric phase of the contraction, your latissimus dorsi is at work.

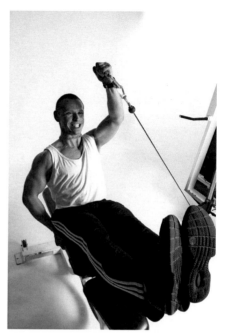

Photo 7.26

Ark's tips:
Remember, warriors, this exercise's value lies in its particular position that forces your muscles to work extra hard. That is why you must make sure you really grab that bench tightly with one hand because this will be the only support for your whole body. You do not want to bend your legs even slightly, and you do not want to round the back. Expand your chest forward and you will really work the back muscles. Keep the muscles in your neck very tight. The small of your back should not touch the back of the bench.

Breathing technique:
Exhale as you pull your arm up and inhale as you return your arm to a position parallel to the floor.

Sports applications:
The essence of this exercise lies in working the core so athletes like gymnasts, dancers, martial artists, and football players will derive great benefit from it.

Modification (for extension-biased persons[34] and persons with shoulder conditions):
Perform a regular Dumbbell Fly on a flat bench, making sure not to lower your arms beyond the level of your horizontally positioned body. Next, place your hands under your tailbone and perform a set of Bicycles with your legs.

CM Dumbbell Shoulder Raises

Difficulty level: I

Caution: If you have back problems, you may be able to perform the exercise modification provided.

Origin: ID

Presenter: Self

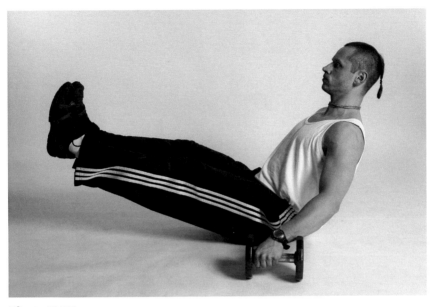

Photo 7.27

Starting position:
Position yourself on a mat. Hold a light dumbbell in both hands using a palm-down grip. Raise both legs straight up in the air to about 40 degrees from the floor and maintain balance. Lean back and arch. Keep the chin up. Your body should form the letter "V" when seen from the side (see Photo 7.27).

Movement:
Simultaneously raise both arms and perform a Dumbbell Lift to about eye level or slightly higher (see Photos 7.28–31). Lower the dumbbells in a similar fashion but without resting them on the mat.

Major muscles involved:
There are quite a few of them here! First of all, by holding the "V" position, you work rectus femoris (upper front thigh), rectus abdominis (especially lower abdominals), and erector spinae (mid- and lower back). These are your stabilizing muscles, and they contract isometrically, or without lengthening and shortening. Second, in the arm, you work the anterior deltoid (front shoulder) and your medial deltoid (middle shoulder). The medial deltoid is the prime mover for the arm.

Ark's tips:
It is crucial to maintain the "V" shape. Otherwise, your back will round and you will create unnecessary strain on the spinal cord.

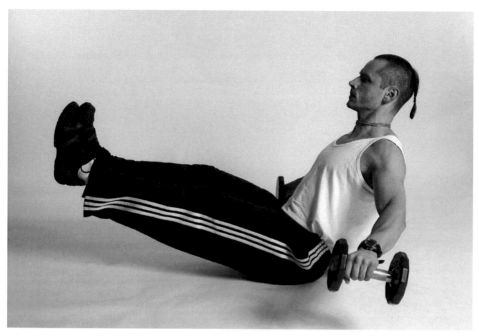

Photo 7.28

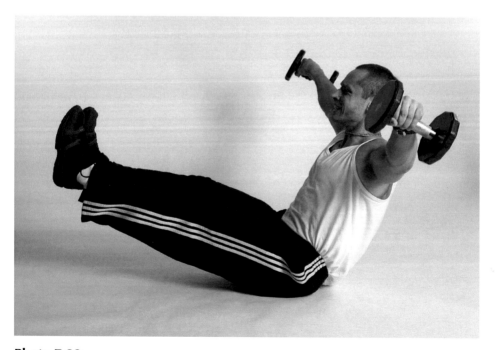

Photo 7.29

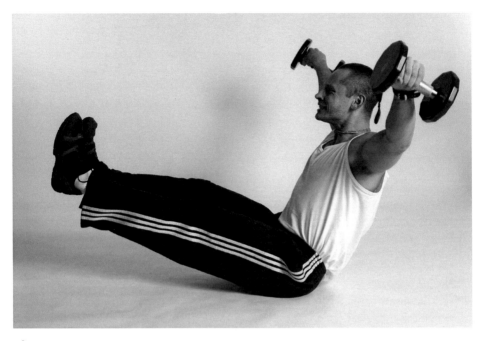

Photo 7.30

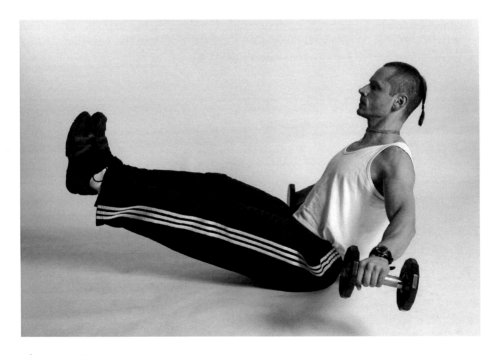

Photo 7.31

Breathing technique:
Exhale as you raise the two dumbbells and inhale as you lower them down.

Sports applications:
Core Master Dumbbell Shoulder Raises force you to contract trunk muscles isometrically (without flexing or extending) in a suspended position. The essence of this exercise lies in working the core so athletes like gymnasts, dancers, martial artists, and football players will derive great benefit from it. There are many sports like boxing, wrestling, or football (linemen who block or hit their opponents) that call for raising of the arms on a consistent basis and, thus, the arm raise will improve endurance of those muscle fibers.

Modification (for extension-biased persons[35]):
See CM Rear Shoulder Circles in this section.

AM Alternated Dumbbell Raise on Incline Bench

Difficulty level: A

Caution: If you have back problems, you may be able to perform the exercise modification provided.

Origin: ID

Presenter: Warrior Greg

Starting position:
Grab two light dumbbells and mount a slanted abdominal bench. Make sure your legs are hooked and secured. Sit up straight, push your chest up, and lean back so that your trunk and legs form at least a 100-degree angle (see Photo 7.32).

Movement:
Begin raising your right and left arms, holding dumbbells in an alternated fashion. Raise them to about eye level and lower them to the side of the bench to your hip (see Photos 7.33–36). Perform at least 10 repetitions for each arm.

Major muscles involved:
First of all, you work rectus abdominis (especially lower abdominals) and erector spinae (mid- and lower back). These are your stabilizing muscles and they contract isometrically, or without lengthening and shortening. Second, in the arm, you work the anterior deltoid (front shoulder). The front shoulder is the prime mover for the arm.

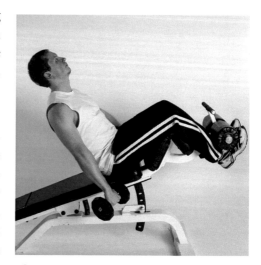

Photo 7.32

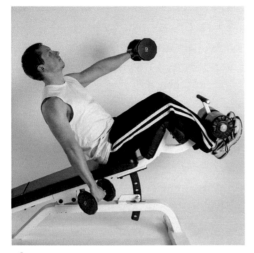

Photo 7.33

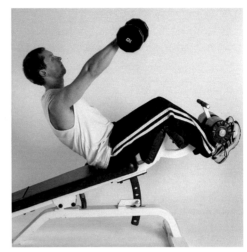

Photo 7.34

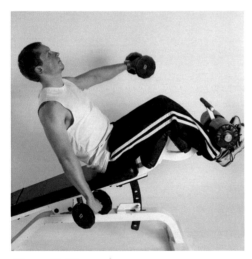

Photo 7.35

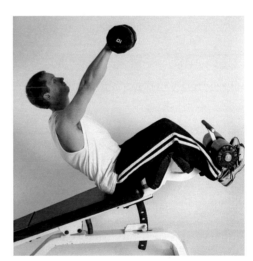

Photo 7.36

Ark's tips:
Complete the raise with one arm (come to a full stop) and then begin raising the other arm.

Breathing technique:
Exhale as you lift the dumbbell and inhale as you lower it.

Sports applications:
The AM Dumbbell Raises force you to contract trunk muscles isometrically (without flexing or extending) in a suspended position. The essence of this exercise lies in working the

core so athletes like gymnasts, dancers, martial artists, and football players will derive great benefit from it. As far as the Shoulder Raise is concerned, we can give the example of *karateka*. The *karateka* is required to keep the hands up on guard at all times, which requires one to constantly maintain a state of isometric contraction in the muscles and execute powerful motions every few seconds. This calls for muscular endurance of fibers in the front shoulder muscle. There are many sports like boxing, wrestling, or football (linemen who block or hit their opponents) that call for raising the arms on a consistent basis and, thus, the arm raise will improve endurance of those muscle fibers.

Modification (for extension-biased persons[36]):
Adjust a flat bench to a recline position and perform the same movement with dumbbells. Next, you can do a set of Crunches or Bicycles on a flat bench (keep your hands under your tailbone).

> Ghatotkacha's Curl/Ab Master Biceps Curl on Incline Bench
>
> Difficulty level: A
>
> Caution: If you have back problems, you may be able to perform the exercise modification provided.
>
> Origin: ID
>
> Presenter: Warrior Rich

Starting position:
Position yourself on a slanted sit-up bench (start out with a low or medium slant and gradually increase it) just as if you were to do a sit-up (sitting position with feet hooked). Hold one medium-weight dumbbell in your right hand. Arch your back so that your chest moves up. Lower your torso to at least a 90-degree angle (measured between upper body and legs). Extend your right arm slightly to

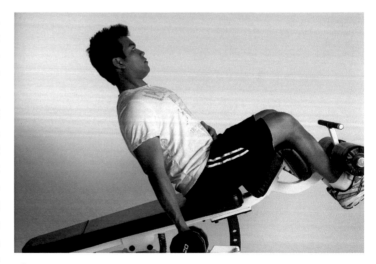

Photo 7.37

the side and below the line of your torso. Bend your left arm and place it on your stomach (see Photo 7.37).

Movement:
While holding the position, execute a regular Dumbbell Curl, flexing the right arm at the elbow until forearm and biceps (front of arm) touch (see Photos 7.38–39). Perform 10 to 12 repetitions and, still holding your torso in that position, switch the dumbbell to your left hand. Repeat on the left side.

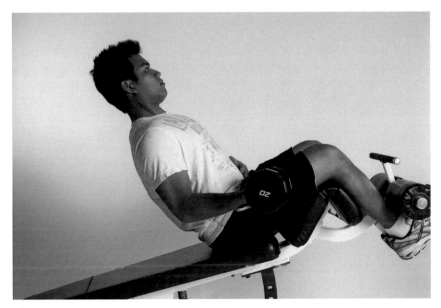

Photo 7.38

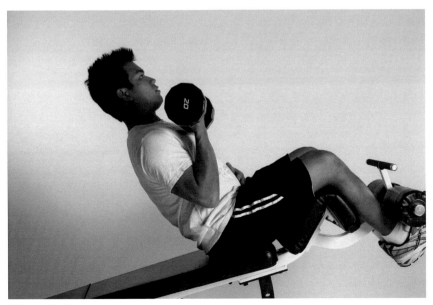

Photo 7.39

Major muscles involved:
The prime mover in the arm is the biceps brachii (front of arm). Stabilizing muscles are rectus abdominis (abdominals), external oblique (sides), as well as erector spinae (lower back).

Ark's tips:
Of course, the greatest advantage of this exercise is not working your biceps, which could be done in so many other, more intense ways, but in creating and maintaining great muscular tension in the abdominal wall and back. Doing a Biceps Curl merely adds to the difficulty of this challenging position in which the core muscles must stay for the duration of the set. Make sure to keep your chest up and, thus, hold your lower back and ab muscles under tension. If your chest caves in and your back rounds, you will be challenging your spine and not the muscles around it.

Breathing technique:
Inhale when extending the arm and breathe out upon flexing.

Sports applications:
Ghatotkacha Curl will work greatly for those athletes whose discipline forces them to maintain intermittent or constant abdominal tension. Gymnasts, circus athletes, and acrobats will benefit from it.

Modification (for extension-biased persons[37]):
Sit in a recline position and perform Biceps Curls. After a set of Curls, get down on the floor and do a set of Bicycles (make sure to keep your hands under your tailbone).

AM Alternated Shoulder Circles

Difficulty level: A

Caution: If you have back problems, you may be able to perform the exercise modification provided.

Origin: ID

Presenter: Warrior Greg

Starting position:
Grab two light dumbbells and mount a slanted abdominal bench. Make sure your legs are hooked and secured. Sit up straight, push your chest up, and lean back so that your trunk and legs form approximately a 145-degree angle (see Photo 7.40).

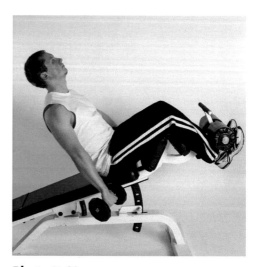

Photo 7.40

Movement:

Using a palm-down or neutral (easier) grip, raise one dumbbell slightly over your head and continue behind your head and to the side and down, making a full circle (see Photos 7.41–44). Then repeat, doing the circle with the other dumbbell. Medium tempo is appropriate for this exercise.

Major muscles involved:

In the midsection, you work rectus abdominis (especially upper abdominals) and erector spinae (mid- and lower back). These are your stabilizing muscles, and they contract isometrically, or without lengthening and shortening. In the arm, you work the anterior

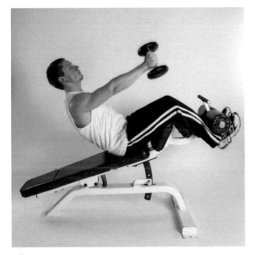

Photo 7.41

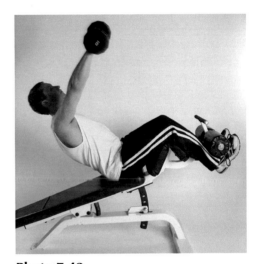

Photo 7.42

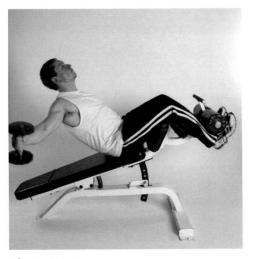

Photo 7.43

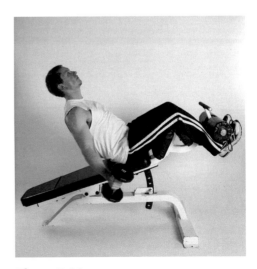

Photo 7.44

deltoid (front shoulder) and your posterior deltoid (rear shoulder). The front shoulder is the prime mover for the arm.

Ark's tips:
Complete the circle with one arm (come to a full stop) and then begin circling the other arm.

Breathing technique:
Exhale as you raise the dumbbell and inhale as you lower it.

Sports applications:
The AM Shoulder Circles force you to contract trunk muscles isometrically (without flexing or extending) in a suspended position. The essence of this exercise lies in working the core and shoulders for endurance. Athletes like gymnasts, dancers, martial artists, and football players will derive great benefit from it. There are many sports like boxing, wrestling, or football (linemen who block or hit their opponents) that call for raising of the arms on a consistent basis and, thus, the arm raise will improve endurance of those muscle fibers.

Modification (for extension-biased persons[38]):
Sit in a recline position and perform the same movement. Next, lie down on a mat with your hands underneath your tailbone and do 15 alternated Bicycles.

Bhima's Core Hold/Under-the-Bar Hold
Difficulty level: S
Origin: ID
Presenter: Self

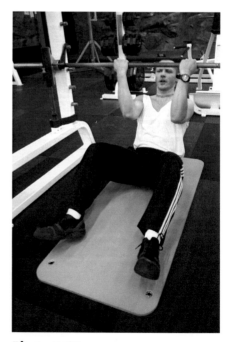

Starting position:
Lower the bar on Smith's Machine so that it is about waist high. Get under the bar and hold it with an undergrip (palms up). Use a medium grip (see Photo 7.45).

Movement:
Commence by tightening up the arms and grab the bar as tightly as you can. Almost simultaneously, tighten up the core muscles very hard and pull yourself off the floor so that you are not touching it with your back or feet. Try to keep the legs as straight as you can. Your body should form the letter "V" when seen from the side (your legs and head are higher than the lower back). Hold the position for at least 15 seconds. See Photos 7.46–50.

Photo 7.45

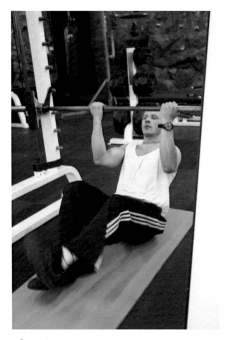
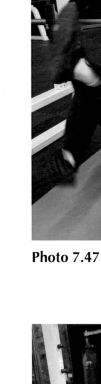

Photo 7.46

Photo 7.47

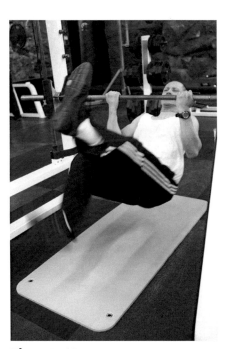
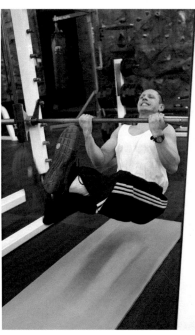

Photo 7.48

Photo 7.49

Major muscles involved:
The Bhima Hold is an isometric exercise, which means that your muscles are neither lengthening nor shortening. They just remain under tension; therefore, all the muscles perform only stabilizing functions. Muscles performing the most amount of work are muscles in the arms, such as biceps brachii (front of arm), brachioradialis (forearms), palmaris longus (forearms), latissimus dorsi (sides of back), and, of course, rectus abdominis (abdominals). You will also work your quadriceps (muscles in front of the thigh).

Ark's tips:
Keep everything as tight as humanly possible. This is only 15 seconds of your life, although it will seem longer. Minimize breathing but focus on maximum tension and keeping your legs straight. Keep your chin down.

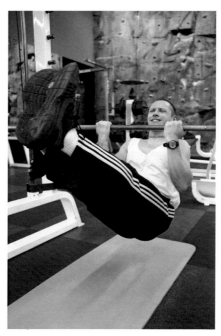

Photo 7.50

Breathing technique:
Try to hold your breath for a major portion of the 15-second period and when you feel you need oxygen, use very short inhalations and exhalations. Alternatively, you could also do a series of longer exhalations and shorter inhalations (much like in karate when you get punched in the stomach, you exhale all the air very forcefully and inhale quickly and then repeat until your state is back to normal).

Sports applications:
Bhima Core Hold is important for all sports that require abdominal strength to produce a good range of motion to lift the legs up high. Therefore, gymnasts and dancers will benefit from the circle kick. Runners can do this exercise to improve their stride length. Kickers in karate, football, and soccer will increase the ability to bring their thighs forward to execute powerful kicks.

The advantage of using an isometric exercise is that it strengthens the muscle in a very specific range of motion. In the case of karate kickers, Bhima Hold will maximize muscle force in the final phase of a front kick and will, therefore, add to the power of the kick. Note, women warriors, that this exercise is very important to eliminate the little extra fat in the lower abs and get a flat tummy.

Core (the core is mainly involved as a prime mover and/or stabilizer)

Dynamic Crunch

Difficulty level: A

Caution: If you have back problems, you may be able to perform the exercise modification provided.

Origin: ID

Presenter: Warrior Greg

Starting position:
Lie on a mat on your back with your hands over the head and your legs shoulder width apart (see Photo 7.51).

Movement:
Crunch up by bending and lifting legs and trunk at the same time. Reach with your hands to your knees. Go back on the mat but only for a split second. Using the kinetic momentum generated from the descend phase of the Crunch, turn on your right side and perform a left side Crunch. Go back down on the mat, but only for a short moment. Turn to the middle and perform a frontal Crunch. Go back down. Turn on the left side and perform a right Crunch. Three Crunches (one front, one left side, one front) will count as one repetition. Then one right, one front, one left (second repetition). Then one front, one right, one front (third repetition). Then one left, one front, one right. And so forth. You can, of course, start on any side and continue in a similar manner reaching eight repetitions. See Photos 7.52–60.

Major muscles involved:
Dynamic Crunch is basically two exercises in combination: a side Crunch, which targets the external obliques (and upper abdominals on both sides) on both sides, and a front Crunch, which targets rectus abdominis (abdominals).

Ark's tips:
Make the movement dynamic enough to generate kinetic momentum to easily turn from side to front and from front to side again. At the same time, be cautious not to increase the range of motion too much as you may hyperextend the spine trying to rock into a Side Crunch and back. Remember, it is not a sit-up (where you raise the trunk to about 45 degrees from the floor or higher), and all you need here is to get the shoulder blades off the mat.

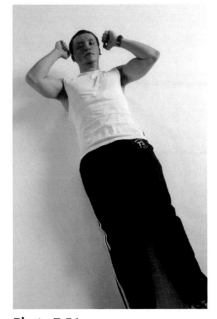

Photo 7.51

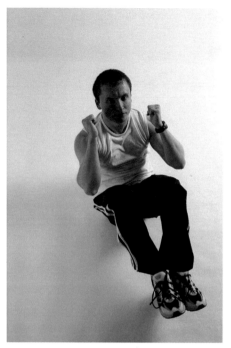

Photo 7.52

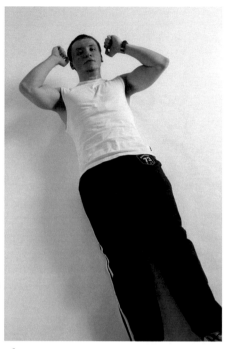

Photo 7.53

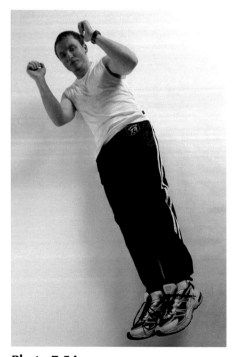

Photo 7.54

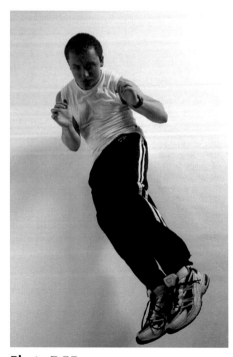

Photo 7.55

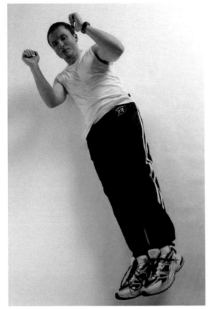

Photo 7.56

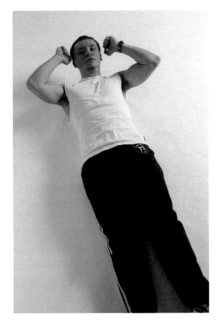

Photo 7.57

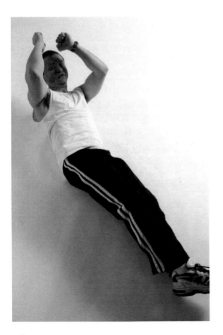

Photo 7.58

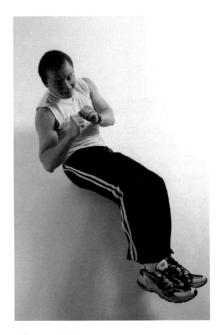

Photo 7.59

Breathing technique:

Quickly exhale as you lift up your trunk and quickly inhale as you get down. Breathe from the core, trying to contract the abdominals maximally with each Crunch pumping the air through them back and forth.

Sports applications:

The movements of the Arjuna Crunch play a role in punching or kicking in the martial arts, and in wrestling as well as in gymnastics (performances on the horizontal bar, pommel horse, cartwheels, etc.). Acrobats who perform many stunts and hand balances can also benefit from the Arjuna Crunch. This exercise is essential for all athletes who throw overhead for distance or force such as javelin athletes, pitchers in baseball, and football quarterbacks. Overhead hitters such as tennis players (serving or smashing), badminton, and racquetball players will also benefit from it. Sports that require one to reach up for maximum height (volleyball, basketball) will benefit from the Arjuna Crunch as well. In the martial arts, such as karate, specifically in blocking and/or receiving a punch in the stomach, a student is required to exhale and contract the abdominal and oblique muscles upon getting hit. This very quick yet deep exhalation and tightening of the core protects one's vital organs and bones, and that's exactly what the Dynamic Crunch trains your body to do.

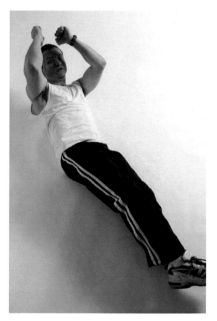

Photo 7.60

Modification (for flexion-biased persons[39]):

Perform a simple Crunch, making sure to lift up only the shoulder blades and not the small of the back. Next, turn on a side and perform a side Crunch, again, making sure to lift up only the shoulder blade.

Isometric Side Crunch

Difficulty level: I

Origin: ID

Presenter: Warrior Kim G.

Starting position:

Lie on a mat on your side (right buttock) and lift up both legs. Keep them straight. Next, straighten out your arms and point them in the direction of the legs. This will facilitate

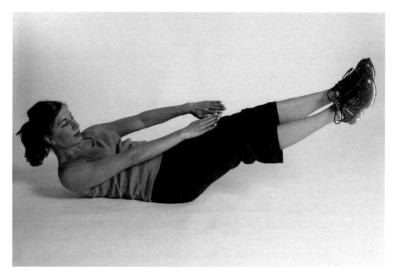

Photo 7.61

contracting the abdominals. Turn your head slightly toward your legs, as if looking in that direction (see Photo 7.61).

Movement:
Without moving your legs, squeeze the left oblique and abdominal muscles. Lift up your trunk so that your right shoulder blade and right side of the back come off the mat. Reach with your joined hands toward the legs (along the left thigh and left knee). Hold a contraction for at least a second, slowly return to your starting position and squeeze again. See Photos 7.62–64. Perform 15 Side Crunches. Switch sides.

Major muscles involved:
When you lie on the right side, you will work the left oblique muscle, rectus abdominis (abdominals), as well as upper quadriceps (thigh) of the right leg and inner thigh of the left leg. When you lie on your left side, the reverse is true, namely the right oblique muscle, the abdominals, upper quadriceps of the left leg, and the inner thigh of the right leg. In addition, the erector spinae muscles (lower back) work considerably in stabilizing the trunk.

Ark's tips:
Try maintaining as much tension in the abdominal wall as you can. Take your time doing this exercise, as its effect lies in prolonging muscle tension. The harder you clench your fists, the more you will be able to contract your abdominals [40] and keep the legs straight.

Breathing technique:
Exhale as you Crunch up, then hold your breath for a second and inhale.

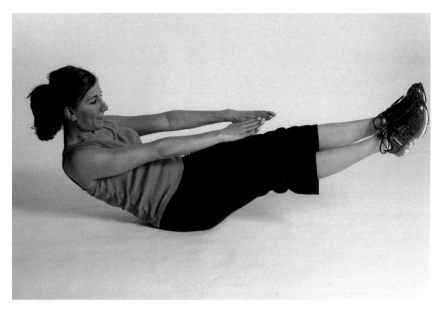

Photo 7.62

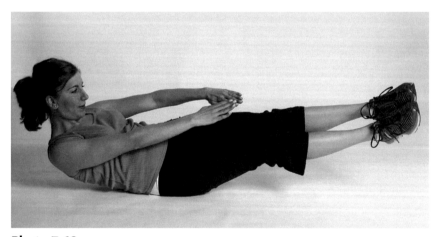

Photo 7.63

Sports applications:
The movements of the Iso Crunch play a role in punching or kicking in the martial arts, and in wrestling as well as in gymnastics (performances on the horizontal bar, pommel horse, cartwheels, etc.). Acrobats who perform many stunts and hand balances can also benefit from the Iso Crunch. The Iso Crunch is also essential for all athletes who throw overhead for distance or force, such as javelin athletes, pitchers in baseball, and football quarterbacks. Overhead hitters such as tennis players (serving or smashing), badminton, and racquetball

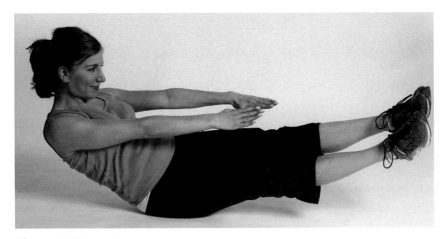

Photo 7.64

players will also benefit from this exercise. Sports that require one to reach up for maximum height (volleyball, basketball) will benefit from the Iso Crunch as well.

Arjuna's Rocking Side Crunch
Difficulty level: I
Origin: IDP
Presenter: Warrior Kim G.

Starting position:
Lie on a mat on your side (right buttock), join both arms, and place them over the head. Lift both legs and keep them straight. Turn your head slightly toward your legs, as if looking in that direction (see Photo 7.65).

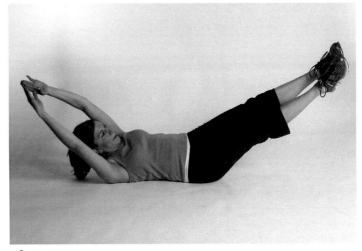

Movement:
Begin rocking back and forth so that each time your upper body comes up, your feet touch the ground and you push yourself off with

Photo 7.65

them (see Photos 7.66–69). Perform 15 rocks on one side and switch.

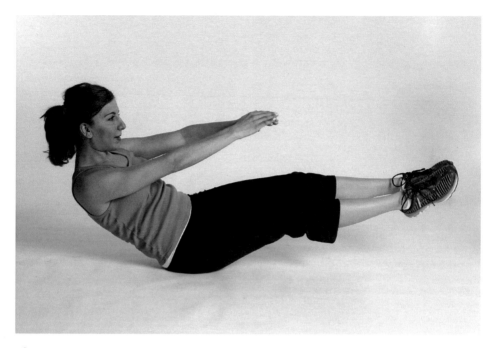

Photo 7.66

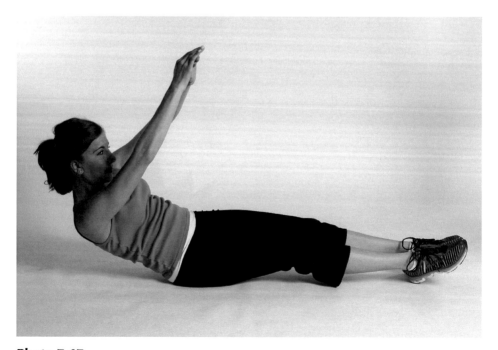

Photo 7.67

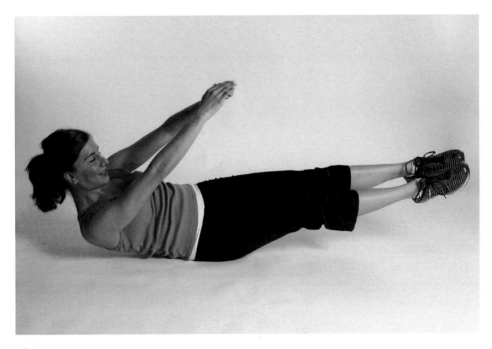

Photo 7.68

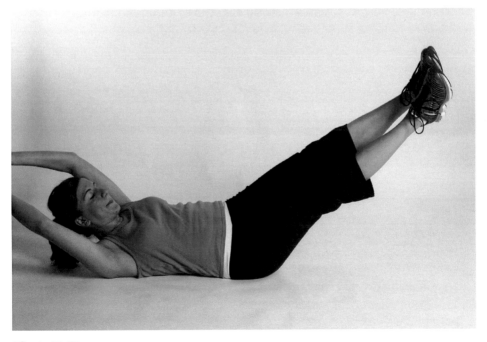

Photo 7.69

Major muscles involved:

When you lie on your right side, you will work the left oblique muscle, rectus abdominis (abdominals), as well as upper quadriceps (thigh) of the right leg and inner thigh of the left leg. When you lie on the left side, the reverse is true, namely right oblique, the abdominals, upper quadriceps of the left leg, and inner thigh of the right leg. The erector spinae muscles (lower back) work considerably in stabilizing the trunk.

Ark's tips:

Maintaining constant high tension in the abdominal wall is the key to doing the Arjuna Crunch correctly. Why? The high tension generated in the abdominal wall will help in contracting the leg and arm muscles, which, in turn, will help in holding the tight position and effective push off. In the Arjuna Crunch, the body works as one unit.

Breathing technique:

Powerfully exhale (as if propelling yourself forward) as your torso comes up from the floor and quickly inhale as the feet come in contact with the floor.

Sports applications:

The movements of the Arjuna Crunch play a role in punching or kicking in the martial arts, and in wrestling as well as in gymnastics (performances on the horizontal bar, pommel horse, cartwheels, etc.). Acrobats who perform many stunts and hand balances can also benefit from the Arjuna Crunch. This exercise is essential for all athletes who throw overhead for distance or force, such as javelin athletes, pitchers in baseball, and football quarterbacks. Overhead hitters such as tennis players (serving or smashing), badminton, and racquetball players will also benefit from it. Sports that require one to reach up for maximum height (volleyball, basketball) will benefit from the Arjuna Crunch as well.

> Hanuman's Circles/Suspended Circles on Dip Stand
>
> Difficulty level: S
>
> Caution: If you have back problems, you may be able to perform the exercise modification provided.
>
> Origin: IDP
>
> Presenter: Self

Starting position:

Climb the dip stand. Make sure your hands are grasping the handles of the stand tightly (your body will be in a vertical position and your arms are bent at the elbows). Tighten up muscles in the core (both back and abdominals) and lift both legs until they are parallel to the floor (see Photo 7.70).

Movement:
Maintain tension in the core muscles by holding a horizontal leg position and perform eight small circles with your legs. You may start the circles clockwise or counterclockwise. Then reverse direction and do another eight circles. See Photos 7.71–76.

Major muscles involved:
This high-tension exercise will target your upper thighs (rectus femoris), as well as rectus abdominis (abdominal muscles).

Ark's tips:
Make sure that you contract muscles in the lower and midback, as this will make it possible to hold this otherwise extremely hard position. Lean forward slightly so that the angle between your torso and legs is a little less than 90 degrees.

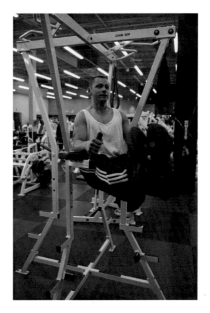

Photo 7.70

Breathing technique:
Perform small exhalations throughout the duration of eight circles and then take a deeper inhalation to begin in the reverse direction.

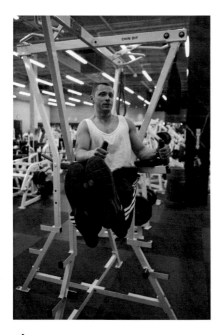

Photo 7.71

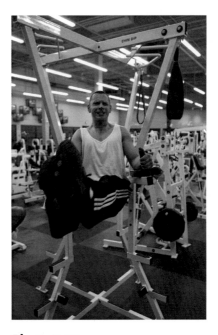

Photo 7.72

Arkadiusz Madej

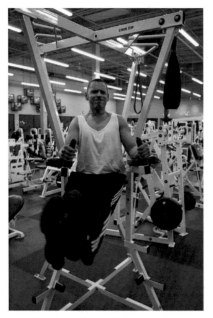

Photo 7.73

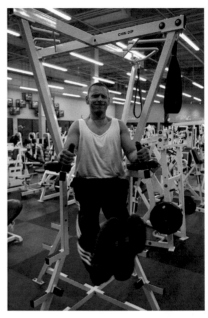

Photo 7.74

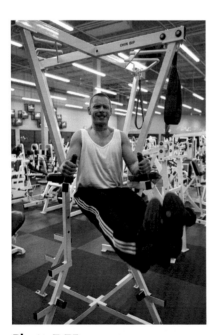

Photo 7.75

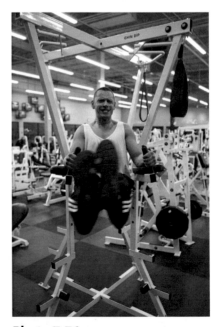

Photo 7.76

Sports applications:
Hanuman Circles are important for all sports that require abdominal strength to produce a good range of motion to lift the legs up high. Gymnasts and dancers will benefit from the circle kick. Kickers in karate, football, and soccer will increase the ability to bring their thighs forward to execute powerful kicks. For martial artists, it is important to be able to receive punches in the stomach while exhaling and Hanuman Circles will help you maintain sufficient tension in the abs.

Modification (for extension-biased persons[41]):
Lie on a mat on your back with your legs straight and hands underneath your tailbone. Next, lift one leg up while the other remains on the floor. Perform 15 small circles just above the floor. Switch legs.

>Dhrstaketu's Jackknives
>
>Difficulty level: A
>
>Caution: If you have back problems, you may be able to perform the exercise modification provided.
>
>Origin: ID
>
>Presenter: Self

Starting position:
Lie down on a mat on your back with your arms extended up and over your head. Your legs should be slightly bent and placed wider than shoulder width (see Photo 7.77).

Movement:
Contract muscles in the core (abdominals, lower, and midback), tighten up thighs and shoulders, and simultaneously raise legs and arms. While going up, make sure you keep the legs straight and your chin down. When your legs and arms get to about 45 degrees off the floor, begin twisting your torso so that your left hand will touch the opposite (right) shin. Return to the position where your midback touches the mat (but shoulder blades are off the floor) and your arms are up. Repeat, this time with your right hand touching the left shin. Perform eight jackknives on each side (16 twists total). See Photos 7.78–85.

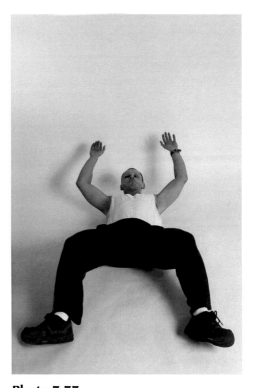

Photo 7.77

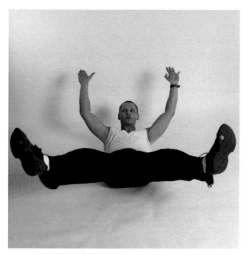

Photo 7.78

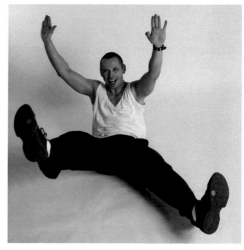

Photo 7.79

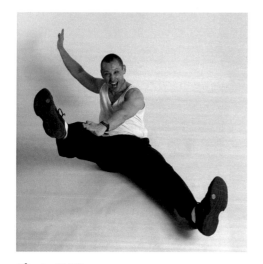

Photo 7.80

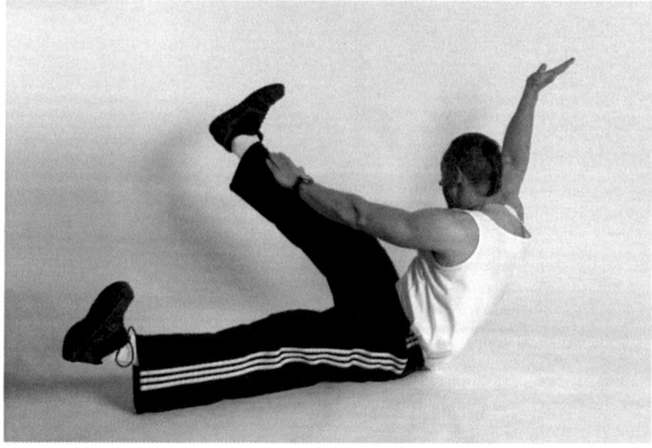

Photo 7.81

Major muscles involved:
A warrior will work the rectus abdominis (abdominals), external obliques (sides), rectus femoris (especially the upper thigh or quadriceps), and posterior deltoids (rear shoulder). Rectus abdominis will be the prime mover in this exercise, and external obliques will assist in the movement. Other muscles perform stabilizing functions.

Ark's tips:
Do not twist too soon as this may put undue stress on your lower spine. Make sure your lower back is off the floor, then go even a little higher and perform the twist (medium or fast tempo).

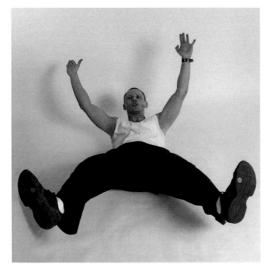

Photo 7.82

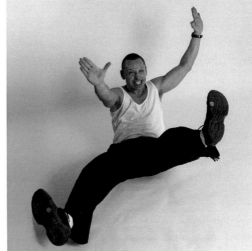

Photo 7.83

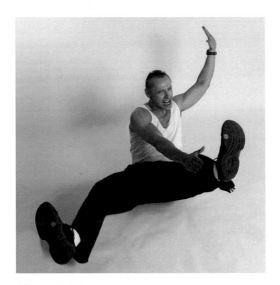

Photo 7.84

Breathing technique:
Exhale through contracted abdominals when going up and finish exhaling upon touching the shin. Inhale quickly going down.

Sports applications:
Dhrstaketu's Jackknives are important for all sports that require abdominal strength to produce a good range of motion to lift the legs up high. Kickers in karate, football, and soccer will

increase the ability to bring their thighs forward to execute powerful kicks. Not only that, but for martial artists, it is important to be able to receive punches in the stomach while exhaling. Dhrstaketu's Jackknives will help you maintain sufficient tension in the abs while twisting. In blocking punches in karate, for instance, you twist inside (*uchi uke* block), which involves contracting oblique and abdominal muscles while contracting the inner thigh muscles. In sweeping kicks such as *soto kaege* (straight leg goes up and inside), you also utilize the very same muscles as in Dhrstaketu's Jackknives, and, therefore, the exercise will prove to be very sport specific. Gymnasts and dancers will benefit from it as well because of the aforementioned factors.

Modification (for people with back conditions):
Lie on a mat on your back with legs straight and hands underneath your tailbone. Next, lift one leg up while the other remains on the floor. Perform 15 leg raises just above the floor. Switch legs.

Lie on a mat on your back with legs straight and hands underneath your tailbone. Next, lift one leg up while the other remains on the floor. Perform 15 small circles just above the floor. Switch legs.

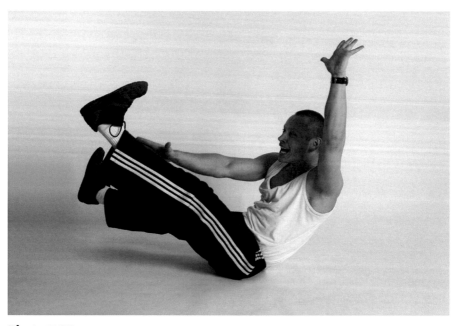

Photo 7.85

Core and lower body (most work in the core involving stabilization, but hip flexors are used as prime movers, legs as assisting stabilizers)

Circle Kick on Vertical Abdominal Bench

Difficulty level: I

Caution: If you have back problems, you may be able to perform the exercise modification provided.

Origin: ID

Presenter: Warrior Susan

Starting position:
Mount a Vertical Abdominal Bench as if for doing leg raises or knee-ups (body almost perpendicular to the floor, back supported by back of chair). Hold on tightly to the side handles of the chair (see Photos 7.86–87).

Movement:
While bending the knees, lift your legs up and straighten them out so that they are parallel to the floor. Remember to go slow. Once straight, lower both legs back to the starting position. (See Photos 7.88–91.) Begin to lift your knees again. Repeat 15 times.

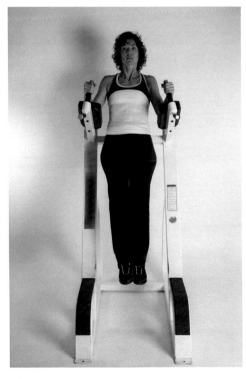

Photo 7.86

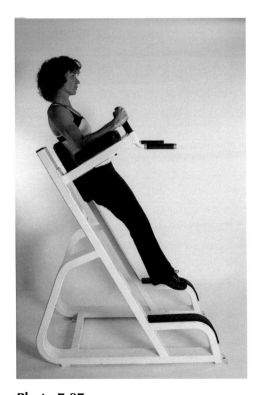

Photo 7.87

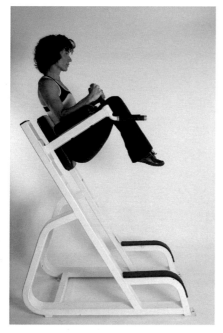

Photo 7.88

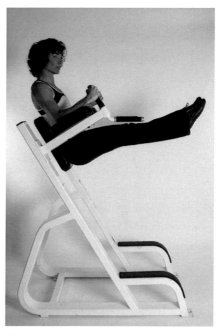

Photo 7.89

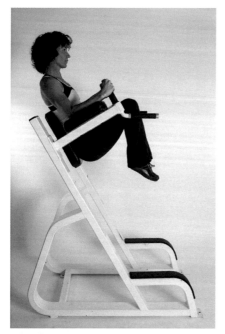

Photo 7.90

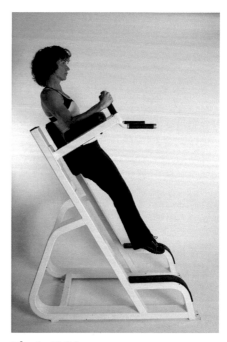

Photo 7.91

Major muscles involved:
In this exercise, you are using your iliopsoas, pectineus (hip flexors), rectus abdominis (abdominals), and rectus femoris (the upper thigh muscles) to lift your knees up. Abdominal muscles such as rectus abdominis are involved to a lesser degree in stabilizing your trunk on your way up and to a greater degree on your way down (with legs straight).

Ark's tips:
Imagine you are leaning backward (although you can't because the seat is stopping you) and push on the back of the seat with your upper back so that you get a good support. Keep muscles in the neck tight. Attempt to straighten out your legs completely before lowering them. You should feel a lot of tension in the quadriceps (thighs).

Breathing technique:
Partially exhale going up and hold your breath when extending your legs out. Once they are straight (parallel to the floor), exhale all the way, while lowering your legs to the starting position.

Sports applications:
Circle Kick is important for all sports that require abdominal strength to produce a good range of motion to lift legs up high. Therefore, gymnasts and dancers will benefit from the Circle Kick. Runners can do this exercise to improve their stride length. Kickers in karate, football, and soccer will increase the ability to bring their thighs forward to execute powerful kicks. Note, female warriors: this exercise is very important to eliminate the little "pouch" in the lower abs and get a flat abdominal wall.

Modification (for extension-biased persons[42]):
Lie on a mat on your back with legs straight and hands underneath your tailbone. Perform 15 Bicycles.

Reverse Circle Kick on Vertical Abdominal Bench

Difficulty level: I

Caution: If you have back problems, you may be able to perform the exercise modification provided.

Origin: ID

Presenter: Warrior Susan

Starting position:
Same as in the previous exercise.

Movement:
Contract abdominal muscles and thigh muscles, and in a controlled medium tempo motion, lift your legs up until they are parallel to the floor. Next, bend your legs at the knees and bring your thighs to your stomach. Lower your legs straight down until they are almost perpendicular to the floor. Repeat 15 times. See Photos 7.92–94.

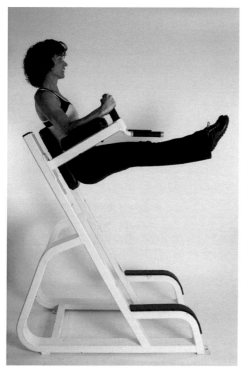 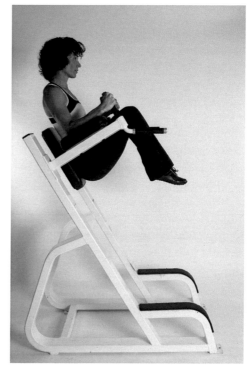

Photo 7.92   **Photo 7.93**

Major muscles involved:
In this exercise, you are using rectus femoris (upper thigh muscles) and rectus abdominis (abdominal muscles) to lift your legs up. Rectus abdominis is the prime mover and rectus femoris, the assisting mover. External obliques stabilize the core to enable you to perform this move. Iliopsoas and pectineus (hip flexors) are used in combination with abdominal muscles to bend your legs and then lower them down.

Ark's tips:
Imagine you are leaning backward (although you can't because the seat is stopping you) and push on the back of the seat with your upper back so that you get a good support. Maintain muscle tension in the neck. Attempt to straighten out your legs completely before bending them to your stomach. You should feel a lot of tension in the quadriceps (thighs).

Breathing technique:
Hold your breath when lifting your legs up and exhale upon bending and bringing them to the stomach. Inhale when lowering your legs down.

Sports applications:
Reverse Circle Kick is important for all sports that require abdominal strength to produce a good range of motion to lift the legs up high. Therefore, gymnasts and dancers will benefit

from the Circle Kick. Runners can do this exercise to improve their stride length. Kickers in karate, football, and soccer will increase the ability to bring their thighs forward to execute powerful kicks. Note, women warriors, that this exercise is very important to eliminate the little extra fat in the lower abs and get a flat tummy.

Modification (for extension-biased persons[43]):
See modification to the previous exercise.

> Roman Ts/Leg Lift with Abduction Adduction on Vertical Abdominal Bench
>
> Difficulty level: I
>
> Caution: If you have back problems, you may be able to perform the exercise modification provided.
>
> Origin: ID
>
> Presenters: Warriors Kim G. and Susan

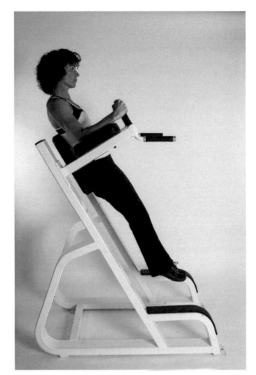

Photo 7.94

Starting position:
Same as in the previous exercise.

Movement:
Contract abdominal muscles and thigh muscles and in a controlled medium tempo motion, lift legs up until they are parallel to the floor. Next, still oscillating in the same horizontal

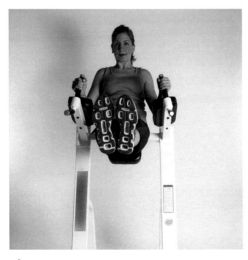

Photo 7.95

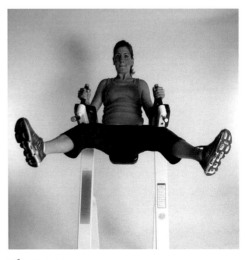

Photo 7.96

plane of motion, open your legs up (at least 70 degrees) and put them together. See Photos 7.95–97. Lower your legs straight down until they are perpendicular to the floor (see starting position). This counts as one repetition. Work up to 15 of them.

Major muscles involved:

In this exercise, you are using rectus femoris (upper thigh muscles) and rectus abdominis (abdominal muscles) to lift your legs up. Rectus abdominis is the prime mover and rectus femoris, the assisting mover. Gracilis and adductor muscles such as adductor longus and magnus (inner thigh) are involved in hip joint adduction, whereas gluteus medius (upper buttock) performs the abduction. External obliques stabilize the core to enable you to perform this move.

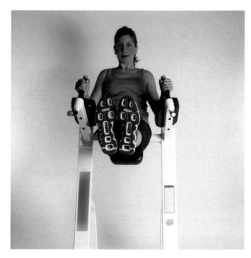

Photo 7.97

Ark's tips:

Imagine you are leaning backward (although you can't because the seat is stopping you) and push on the back of the seat with your upper back so that you get a good support. Maintain muscle tension in the neck. Keep the core as tight as you can. This will enable you to maintain your legs in a position parallel to the floor.

Breathing technique:

Exhale as you lift up your legs. Then inhale upon abducting and exhale upon adduction and lowering the legs. Once in the down position, take a deeper breath. Repeat the same breathing pattern.

Sports applications:

Roman Ts are important for all sports that require abdominal strength to produce a good range of motion to lift the legs up high. Gymnasts and dancers will benefit from the Roman T. Kickers in karate, football, and soccer will increase the ability to bring their thighs forward to execute powerful kicks.

In addition, hip abduction is crucial in lateral movement. The examples are many (soccer, football, handball, ice hockey, tennis, etc.). Leg abduction is also important in shifting body weight in hitting and throwing. We may mention sports like boxing, karate, javelin throwing, and golf (swinging the club). Hip joint adduction is the key in sports that require maneuvering such as lacrosse, soccer (e.g., kicking with the inside of the foot when passing the ball), volleyball, basketball, etc. It will help in doing turns, crossover steps, and also shifting weight from one foot to another.

Modification (for extension-biased persons[44]):
Lie on a mat on your back with your legs straight and hands underneath your tailbone. Next, lift one leg up while the other remains on the floor. Perform 15 horizontal leg moves and switch legs.

Combinations (the legs are mainly involved as stabilizing muscles, but the arms are prime movers)

Balarama's Circles/Hanging from Bar Shoulder Circle

Difficulty level: I

Origin: IDP

Presenter: Warrior Bill

Starting position:
Grab onto a horizontal bar (you could use the Smith Machine) or handle with one hand. Hold a medium-size dumbbell in the other. Squat down to 90 degrees (the angle measured between your calf and back of the thigh). Lean back and make sure your torso is perpendicular to the floor (it will be easier to do since you are using support). See Photo 7.98.

Movement:
Using a palm-down grip, raise the dumbbell slightly over your head and continue to the side and down making a full circle (see Photos 7.99–104). Repeat 15 times and switch hands.

Major muscles involved:
Since you are squatting, you are using the same muscles as in other exercises that utilize squats (e.g., Samurai Squats in Chapter II, or Bhima's Shoulder Rover below). All leg muscles are at work, as well as core muscles (abdominals, lower back), stabilizing the position. In the arm, you work your anterior deltoid (front shoulder) and, depending on how far back you draw the circle, your posterior deltoid (rear shoulder). The front shoulder is the prime mover for the arm.

Ark's tips:
Lean back to ensure full stress of the leg muscles. Maintain a slow to medium tempo.

Breathing technique:
Exhale as you raise the dumbbell and inhale as you lower it.

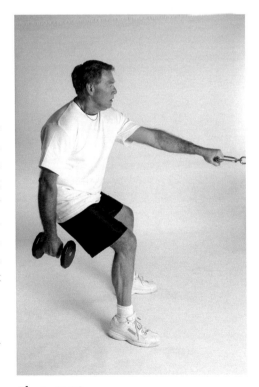

Photo 7.98

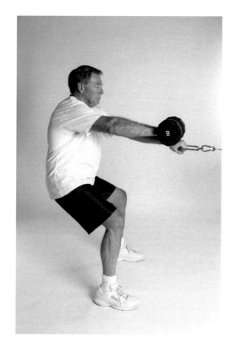

Photo 7.99

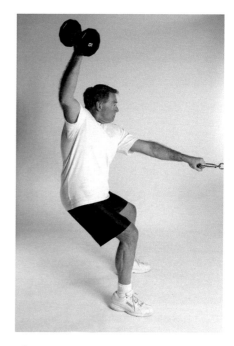

Photo 7.100

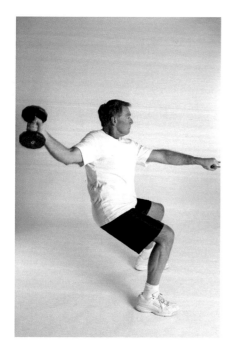

Photo 7.101

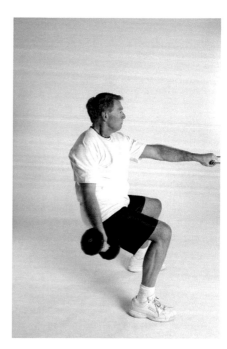

Photo 7.102

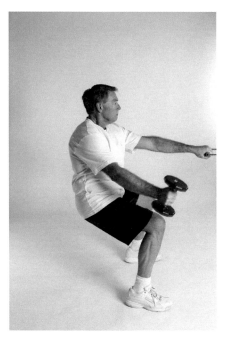

Photo 7.103

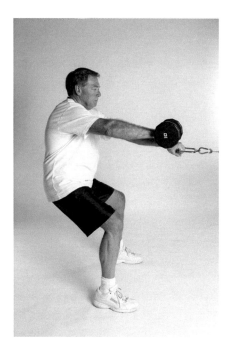

Photo 7.104

Sports applications:

Any sport that requires muscle endurance in the leg and shoulder area will benefit from Samurai Squats. Take karate, for example. In sparring matches or fighting, the *karateka* is supposed to keep a low stance with knees bent to facilitate mobility and agility (everything depends on footwork and maintaining the right distance from the opponent). As far as arm work is concerned, the *karateka* is required to keep the hands up on guard at all times (in Kyokushin karate, you keep them up even when you deliver a kick), which requires one to constantly maintain a state of isometric contraction in the muscles and execute powerful motions every few seconds. This calls for muscular endurance of certain muscle fibers. There are many sports that call for raising of the arms on a consistent basis, and thus the arm raise will improve endurance of those muscle fibers.

Bhima's Shoulder Rover

Difficulty level: I

Origin: ID

Presenter: Warrior Bill

Starting position:

Pick up two medium-weight dumbbells. Stand in a horse riding stance, that is, with the legs bent at the knees and back perpendicular to the floor (straight). Bend both arms holding two dumbbells and raise them so that they are slightly over your shoulders (but not resting on them). The grip used should be neutral (palms of hands facing one another), and your arm should form a right angle between biceps and forearm. See Photo 7.105.

Movement:

Aiming straight ahead in a slow motion, punch your left fist forward (doing so, you may or may not want to twist your wrist, depending on how specific to your sport you would like the exercise to be). See Photo 7.105. As the hand is almost fully extended (but with slight room in the elbow joint), begin lowering it down slowly until the back of your arm (triceps) or its side touches the left pectoralis (chest). Next, bring it back up in a curling motion (shortened Biceps Curl). See Photos 7.106–109. Do the same for the right side. That counts as one repetition. Perform 15 of them on each side (30 circles).

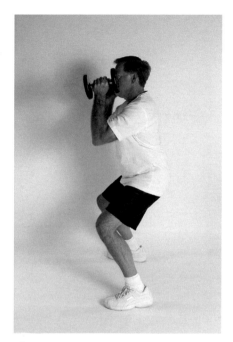

Photo 7.105

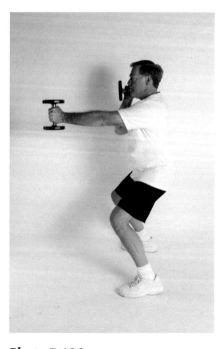

Photo 7.106

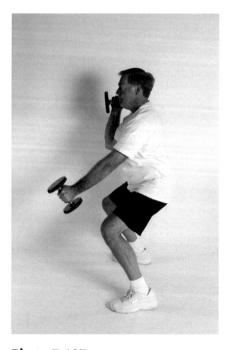

Photo 7.107

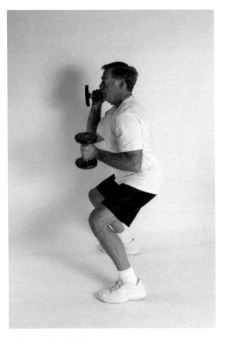

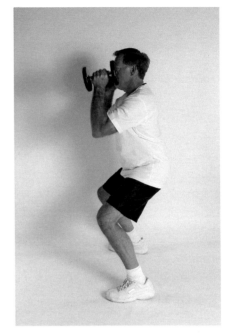

Photo 7.108   **Photo 7.109**

Major muscles involved:
All of the muscles in the legs and torso are at work because you are squatting in a horse riding stance, which involves the legs, and stabilizing for the Rover motion. In the arms, you work the anterior deltoid (front shoulder) and biceps brachii (front of arm).

Ark's tips:
Maintain a slow tempo and consciously contract core and arm muscles. Remember, faster—as you may already have learned—is not always better.

Breathing technique:
Hold your breath as you launch the arm forward and begin exhaling as your arm is straightening out. By the time your arm is halfway lowered, you should have completed the exhalation. Start inhaling again. By the time your arm is back up in a neutral position, you should be ready to hold your breath and exhale again.

Sports applications:
The Bhima Rover will prove successful in developing maximum strength (see the chapter on different kinds of strength) for your punches. Therefore, sports like boxing (uppercut), wrestling, judo, or various martial arts will benefit from this exercise. In addition, football linemen may be able to strengthen their arms for blocking or hitting an opponent. Bhima Rover will help all those who use underhand throws or hits. We may mention here bowling, softball (pitching), handball (underhand shot), hockey (preparation for different shots), etc.

Garuda Shoulder Lift/Low Cable Shoulder Raise on One Foot
Difficulty level: A
Origin: IDP
Presenter: Warrior Kim D.

Starting position:
Set an adjustable pulley station to the lowest notch and a relatively low weight (10–15 pounds). Grasp the handle of the pulley with your right hand and turn your left shoulder to the station so that the right arm is away from the pulley station. Stand on your left foot and bend over so that your trunk is almost parallel to the floor. Both legs should be kept as straight as possible. The right arm holding the handle should be slightly bent. The left arm is raised and kept high for added balance. See Photo 7.110.

Movement:
Tighten up your lower back and the muscles in the supporting leg. Then pull your right arm away from the pulley and up until it becomes aligned with your torso. Keep the right arm straight. Use a medium tempo for this exercise. See Photos 7.111–112.

Major muscles involved:
The supporting muscles of the leg you stand on are: gluteus maximus (buttock), gastrocnemius (calf muscle), and various muscles of the foot (you will feel how intensely they work). Back extensors (lower back), as well as external oblique muscles (sides) are at work to stabilize your trunk for executing the Garuda Shoulder Lift. The prime mover for the arm is the posterior deltoid (back shoulder), and its assistant is trapezius (upper back).

Ark's tips:
The key to doing this exercise correctly and effectively is keeping all muscles tight (especially your core and legs) and balancing your body. Take your time, go slower, focus on breathing.

Breathing technique:
Exhale as you lift the arm and inhale upon bringing it back down. Remember, speed of your breathing must be synchronized with the speed of your movement.

Sports applications:
Garuda Shoulder Lift trains lower body and core muscles needed in weight lifting (e.g., clean and snatch, dead lift), running (e.g., pushing off), gymnastics, trampolining, as well as diving.

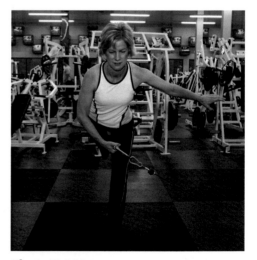

Photo 7.110

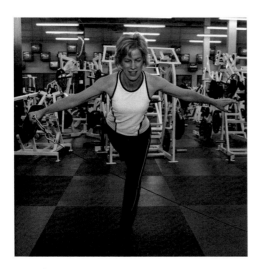

Photo 7.111

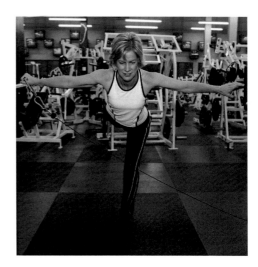

Photo 7.112

The rear shoulder action will be useful in tennis, racquetball, badminton, baseball (e.g., batting), archery (pulling back action), gymnastics (e.g., iron cross), and any rowing sport.

Karate Punch

Difficulty Level: I

Caution: If you have back problems, you may be able to perform the exercise modification provided.

Origin: K

Presenter: Warrior Kim D.

Starting position:
Lie on a mat on your stomach with your left hand out in front of you and the other alongside your body. Tighten up muscles in the back, in the arms, and lift up the upper body and legs so that the chest, arms, and knees do not touch the mat. Bend your right arm and make a fist. Make a fist with the other hand too. See Photo 7.113.

Movement:
Punch forward with your right arm as you withdraw the left arm. Make sure you look up and punch straight ahead. Then punch forward with the left arm as you withdraw the right. See Photos 7.114–115. This counts as one repetition and you should do 15 of them (30 punches). Maintain a rapid tempo and pause briefly after each punch.

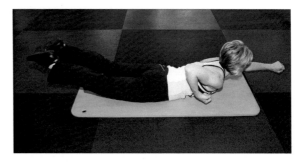

Photo 7.113

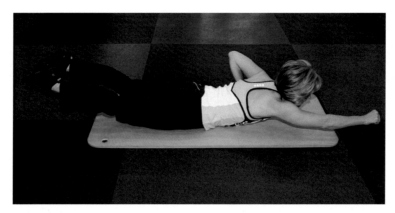

Photo 7.114

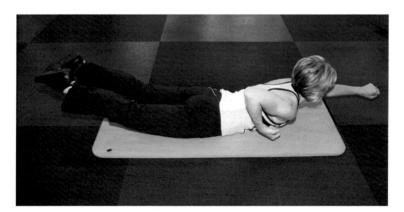

Photo 7.115

Major muscles involved:
The stabilizing muscles acting here are erector spinae (lower back), gluteus maximus (buttocks), rectus abdominis (abdominals), as well as external obliques (sides). The anterior deltoid (front shoulder) is the prime mover for the arm, and the posterior deltoid (rear shoulder) is the antagonist mover (it withdraws the arm after the punch).

Ark's tips:
Tense up as you finish each punch, then relax slightly, maintaining tension mostly in the back, and punch again. Look at your punching fist.

Breathing technique:
Synchronize breathing with your punching. As you punch, exhale rapidly, pause for a second, and inhale, punch, and exhale again. Exhaling is always faster than inhaling.

Sports applications:
Swimmers can benefit from Karate Punch because it uses the same muscles in a very similar way. Wrestlers (e.g., bridge) and judokas (takedowns and throws) will benefit as well. Karate Punch is a great exercise for improving posture in general. Proper posture is crucial in sports like gymnastics, ballet, and dancing. Rowers rely on strong lower back muscles. High jumpers and volleyball players will benefit from this exercise as they need to jump, reach for the ball, and arch their backs.

Modification (for extension-biased persons[45]):
Lie down but with both hands alongside your body and resting on the mat, then contract the muscles in the back and your butt. Hold the contraction for at least 2 seconds. Repeat 15 times.

Appendix A

WHY IS VEGETARIANISM HEALTHIER?

Everyone, and especially Krishna warriors, should eat nutritious foods. You feel and are what you eat.

Vegetarianism is the most suitable diet for every human being, especially those involved in intense physical training. Human beings are not biologically suited to eating meat. Human teeth, like those of plant-eating animals, are suited to grinding and chewing rather than ripping and tearing, as is necessary with flesh-eaters. Meat-eating animals usually swallow their food without chewing it. Therefore, they do not possess molars. Neither are their jaws capable of moving from side to side in a chewing motion.

Human hands are not equipped with sharp claws, but instead, have opposable thumbs necessary for those who must harvest their foods (4 Prabhupada 1).

Meat requires strong digestive juices to digest it if it is not to rot in the stomach. Humans and other plant-eating entities produce acid one-twentieth the strength of the stomach acids found in carnivores. Carnivores also have short intestinal tracts; meat rots quickly and

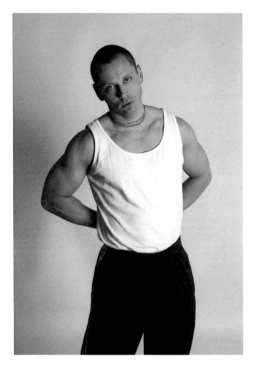

Do you really need to support so much violence committed every day to those little creatures that live along with us? Or is it just that your taste buds like animal corpses, and you cannot conquer them?

must be moved through the body before it becomes toxic to the eater. Carnivores possess alimentary canals only three times the length of their bodies. Humans and other plant-eating beings have long alimentary canals; their intestines are 12 times their body length. The bodies of humans who eat meat are stressed by having to move the meat through such long intestines.

The toxins produced in the body tend to alter the natural metabolism, which is made for the digestion of carbohydrates. Diabetes may result. Furthermore, so much energy going to digestion tends to divert life energy from other functions, including thinking. And those who consume meat absorb into their bodies many toxic wastes that would otherwise be expelled from the animal's body as urine (4 Prabhupada 3).

The kidneys are responsible for the elimination of toxins. Meat eaters strain their kidneys, overloading them with poisonous substances produced during the body's attempt to digest meat. The kidneys of even moderate meat eaters do three times more work than the kidneys of their vegetarian counterparts. Young people can cope with the added stress, but as people age, the risk of kidney disease and renal failure becomes greater (4 Prabhupada 3).

Meat-eating humans also struggle to deal with excessive animal fats. Natural carnivores can metabolize almost unlimited amounts of cholesterol and fat without negative effects, but humans cannot. When over a period of years an excess of uneliminated fats builds up, arteries harden and stroke or heart attacks becomes imminent (4 Prabhupada 3-4).

There is also a higher chance of contracting colon cancer among meat eaters again, because of the toxic wastes moved to the digestive system after digestion. Aside from the natural toxins produced by undigested meat, factory-produced meat contains preservatives, antibiotics, and the remains of untreated animal diseases. Meat is often loaded with DDT, arsenic (used in cattle food as a growth stimulant), sodium sulfate (gives meat a "fresh" red color), and DES (a carcinogen)[46] (Rosen 9).

For many people, the single most compelling evidence against meat eating is the well-documented correlation between meat consumption and heart disease. America has the highest rate of meat consumption in the world, and in America, one out of every two persons will die of heart-related complications. Such diseases are lower in nations where meat consumption is low (Rosen 10).

What about the need for dietary protein? Many powerful animals get their protein from vegetable sources—think of elephants, bulls, and rhinoceri. Each of these animals is both powerful and vegetarian. Flesh foods contain no amino acids that cannot be obtained from plant foods eaten in a proper combination.

The famous Mr. Universe bodybuilder Bill Pearl[47] confirms (Pearl 34), "You do not need meat for protein. About half of the world's population does not eat meat for religious or other reasons. There are also large groups of people in the United States, such as Seventh Day Adventists, who do not eat meat at all—and display much better health than the average American. . . .

"Where do they obtain their protein? The answer is simple: proteins are a part of virtually every natural food available to man. Every plant, every seed, and every fruit contains some protein. It is virtually impossible not to obtain enough protein in any diet of natural foods.

"The long-held belief that meat proteins are superior to vegetable proteins has been disproved. Recent research has demonstrated that animal proteins in any amounts have a detrimental effect on health, and that vegetable proteins, formerly believed to be incomplete or inferior to animal proteins, are actually biologically as good or better than animal proteins. . . . You also do not need meat protein for strength."

The idea that large amounts of protein are required for energy and strength is a myth. When proteins are digested, they break down into amino acids, which the body uses for growth and tissue replacement. The body itself can synthesize all but eight of the 22 amino acids. These eight essential amino acids are found in abundance in nonflesh foods (4 Prabhupada 8).

Asked what his diet consists of when training for Mr. Universe contests and what the best protein supplement is, Bill Pearl replies, "my morning and afternoon meals will almost be all eggs and some fresh fruit and raw vegetables . . . to keep the fat content down, we will keep backing off the yolks. For my evening meal, I will have some type of meat substitute and fresh vegetables and maybe some cooked vegetables and some type of fruit like cantaloupe, watermelon, or honeydew. . . .

"The best type of protein a person can ingest [meat substitute] is a milk and egg protein concentrate. The protein efficiency ration in milk and eggs is the highest you can possibly get. The manufacturers of milk and egg protein concentrates have already extracted the protein and amino acids from the milk [e.g., whey protein] . . . So meat is no more than another substance to put in our body, and what little bit of protein and carbohydrates and minerals that are there, your body will extract it and use it like any other food. Meat is definitely not the secret to bodybuilding (Weis 1–2)."

When we consume foods from the plant kingdom, we combine our assimilation of amino acids with the assimilation of other essential nutrients for proper anabolism, such as carbohydrates, vitamins, minerals, enzymes, hormones, chlorophyll, etc. Besides, the body uses protein as a last resort; when we don't consume enough carbohydrates, the body will use protein for energy. The body's main source of energy comes from carbohydrates (Rosen 5–6).

When we eat too much protein, the body's energy capacity is reduced. Physical tests show that vegetarians are able to perform physical tasks two to three times longer than meat eaters before exhaustion sets in. They also fully recover from fatigue up to five times faster (Rosen 5–6). Says Bill, who won the professional Mr. Universe in 1971—at the age of 41—without the use of steroids and as a vegetarian: "With each succeeding year on the diet (lacto-ovo vegetarian), I've felt better. I'm more healthy; I can train with more energy (Bill Pearl 'the Vegetarian Bodybuilder').

"Regarding your question about the grams of protein per pound of muscle bodyweight, I have done studies on this, and I've read more on protein that you can shake a stick at. If you're consuming half a gram of protein per pound of muscle bodyweight regardless of how hard you train, that's all you need for repair and muscle growth; that's it. Any more than that will either be stored as fat, or you can consume as fuel. So if a person is taking 400 or 500 grams of protein a day, they're wasting their money and would be better off eating Hershey's candy bars, because they can be digested quicker (Weis 5)."

Some people may already know that the current position of the American Dietetic Association recommends a meatless diet as healthier and adequate when appropriately planned. (See the November 1993 issue of their journal.) Also, the *Dietary Guidelines for Americans*, issued by the U.S. Department of Agriculture and Health and Human Services, represents the current federal policy on the role of dietary factors in health and disease prevention.

"Vegetarian diets are consistent with the Dietary Guidelines and can meet Recommended Dietary Allowances for nutrients. Protein is not limiting in vegetarian diets as long as the variety and amounts of foods consumed are adequate." (This report was issued in September 1995 [Rosen 7].)

ETHICAL CONSIDERATIONS

A warrior does not wish to cause undue suffering to any living entity; no gentleman would want to do that. Slaughtering an animal is painful for the animal and causes it suffering. On the physical and emotional levels, both animals and humans are "feeling" creatures. Irrespective of whether we kill them slowly or quickly, animals suffer.

We are each given a material body and a life span. To cut another entity's life span short without good cause is sinful. Says Bill Pearl, "I've become more concerned with my fellow man and the other inhabitants I share the planet with. . . . I have now been a vegetarian for almost 20 years. We have not fish, fowl, or red meat in our diet. Yet I can still carry the same amount of muscle as I did in winning my four Mr. Universe titles. People can't believe it. They think that to have big muscles you have to eat meat—it's a persistent and recurring myth. But take it from me, there's nothing magic about eating meat that's going to make you a champion bodybuilder (Bill Pearl 'the Vegetarian Bodybuilder')."

The majority of biologists consider consciousness only in terms of behavior. They do not look at behavior as a symptom of a spiritual presence in the entity. This is called material reductionism. Many biologists and other such scientists are atheists and deny the existence of God, the soul, and the spiritual world. Most do not consider animals "sentient." That is, they think there is no real difference between stones and dogs. Whatever sensation an animal experiences can never be compared to human experience. Scientists use this argument to justify laboratory experiments on animals, as well as meat eating.

However, this argument cannot stand up to reason. If we examine animals, we will see that they are characterized by all the same traits as humans. This is how we determine that they are alive. Why do animals being led to slaughter struggle? Stones do not struggle when they are being brought to destruction because they are not alive.

What is the difference between stones (or dead bodies) and living entities? Animals eat and people eat; animals sleep and people sleep; animals bleed and people bleed; animals reproduce and people reproduce. Similarly, both animals and humans experience pain and pleasure. Can we place a value on the actual degree of an animal's suffering when compared to a human's? That doesn't seem logical.

Because our society has learned to devalue animal suffering, it does not use anesthetics to ease the pain animals may feel. Cruelty is common in stockyards. Sick and injured animals may live for days before being slaughtered. Factory farming is horrendously cruel. In factory henhouses, a number of hens are raised in 12 × 18 inch cages. The hens are driven mad by the lack of space, and they attempt to peck each other to death. Farmers then de-beak the birds, a painful process in itself. The hens are kept as long as they lay a certain number of eggs in a week. If they fail to meet their quota, they are culled and slaughtered.

Although most eggs go unfertilized, roosters are allowed to fertilize a certain number of eggs to keep up the production of hens. Male chicks are disposed of at hatching by "chick-pullers." Up to 500,000 male chicks are born in the U.S. daily. They are culled from the females, then placed in plastic bags where they often suffocate or are crushed under other chicks. Some remain alive long enough to be ground up as livestock feed or fertilizer.

Most countries have inhumane laws regarding animal slaughter. Those who are interested should inform themselves of these laws (Rosen 4–5). Animal killing, regardless of the animal's level of development, breeds callousness, insensitivity toward other beings, sadism, and proves a lack of reverence for life.

ECONOMICS AND ENVIRONMENTAL ETHICS

There is much to support a vegetarian diet for those who care to inform themselves. Other points to consider when thinking about the impact your diet has on the earth are economics, world hunger, spiritual teachings found in all faiths (the Bible teaches, "Thou shalt not kill"[48]), and the science presented in the Vedas (such as the teaching that all living entities possess souls and should not be treated with violence, etc.).

From the economical point of view, consider the following statistics: One thousand acres of soybeans yields 1,124 pounds of protein. One thousand acres of corn yields 1,009 pounds of protein. One thousand acres of rice yields 938 pounds of protein. One thousand acres of wheat yields 1,043 pounds of protein. One thousand acres of grains or legumes, when fed to a steer, yields only 125 pounds of protein. The farmland is left barren as well. One acre used to raise a steer will yield only about 1 pound of protein. The same area planted with soybeans yields 17 pounds of protein. It has been estimated that raising livestock consumes eight times more water than growing vegetables or grains because the cattle drink and the crops that feed them must also be watered (Rosen 8).

Another piece of evidence makes us aware that meat consumption produces methane, which is one of the four greenhouse gases contributing to global warming. For example, the 1.3 billion cattle in the world produce one-fifth of all the methane emitted in the atmosphere.

Most people know that the world's priceless rainforests are being destroyed day by day as the lumber and meat industries transform them into giant pastures to provide cheap beef (Rosen 8).

AESTHETIC FACTORS

Many of us are aware that the odor of animal and fish carcasses are horrible and are tolerated only with the help of intoxication to dull the senses. People often dress meat with spices and sauces, and cook it so that it is finally accepted by the body without repulsion. Most people would not dare to eat raw meat. What if they had to personally slaughter the animal first? Most children have to be forced to eat fish. On the other hand, dishes prepared from the plant kingdom are colorful, pleasing to the eye, delightful to smell, and delicious on the tongue.

In conclusion, honest spiritual warriors have to admit that Mother Nature does not force us to build slaughterhouses and eat meat. Meat may be consumed as a last resort—during times of starvation. Vegetarianism is the only nutritious way for civilized humans to eat. For those pursuing a holistic path of life, vegetarian nutrition is a must. For those interested in further study, I recommend they read the comprehensive book, *Diet for Transcendence,* by Steven Rosen.

Appendix B

CHANNELING SEXUAL DESIRE

The proper use of sexual energy is not only beneficial, but also varied and invaluable. It is essential to Krishna warriors.

Many of us may agree that the whole world revolves around sexual desire, and not only in the human species of life. A man wants to attract and possess a suitable woman and vice versa. Then families and societies are developed based on this desire and with whatever helps in its functioning. Sexual desire is directly related to semen.[49]

Semen is a valuable fluid. People who control their drive for sense enjoyment (especially their sexual drive) control their semen. As a result, they live longer, look younger, and retain their reproductive potential well into old age. Professor Charles E. Brown-Séquard, a French physiologist and neurologist who is often considered the "father of endocrinology," discov-

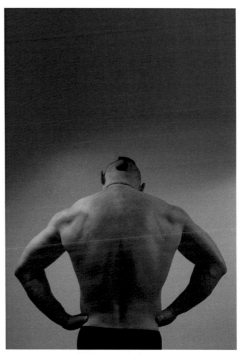

It is so difficult sometimes . . .

ered that voluntary saving of semen within one's body strengthens a man and is conducive to long life. This is because semen is returned to the body, which acts as a tonic for the nervous system (Danavir 69).

Not only that, but to spend semen unwisely spoils the possibility of understanding spiritual truth and reaching a full human potential. When we don't expend semen unnecessarily, it rises to the brain and nourishes brain tissue. Continence increases memory, determination, intelligence, and physical strength (5 Prabhupada 237).

We find much evidence from the field of psychiatry that there is a strong relationship between the sex glands and the brain (Danavir 17). We learn that both the brain and the sex organs extract the same substances from the blood to produce their fluids (22). "No two organs show greater similarity in their lecithin, cholesterin, and phosphorus contents as the semen and the brain (22)." Seminal discharge involves a sudden withdrawal of calcium, lecithin, and other substances necessary for the normal functioning of the nervous system

(19). The gray matter of the brain contains 17 percent lecithin, which is crucial to higher intellectual processes. The greater the purity in which lecithin is found, the higher the intelligence (21).

The Ayurveda, ancient medical scriptures of India, gives a detailed look at *shukra* (semen, or in females, the ovum). Semen is one of the seven structural elements (*dhatus*) of the body, which also include lymph, blood, muscle, fat, marrow, and bone. The body is built and maintained by these seven *dhatus*. We obtain these substances from the food we digest (Adhikari 7). (Note that it is not what we *eat* that strengthens the body, but what we digest. Thus, absorption of food is as important as eating the right food.)

Once the food is digested, it forms all seven substances, one after the other. When lymph forms, blood forms, and from blood, muscle. Semen is the last to be formed and is the most important, because it contains the previous six substances. Therefore, it is known as virya, "vital essence." When semen is lost, the other structures are lost with it (7).

Prof. Eugen Steinach, an eminent physiologist, corroborated this in his experiments which showed that the internal secretions of the sex glands are absorbed into the bloodstream and, thereafter, pass mostly to the brain and spinal cord, where they are stored (Danavir 20). Therefore, a warrior should be aware that his semen does not only remain in his reproductive organs but pervades his entire body. It radiates energy and helps form the aura.

The Ayurveda offers the following calculation: When considering measuring purposes, one pound of food equals 100 cubic centimeters. Ten cc of lymph forms from 1 pound of food. Five cc of blood is formed from the 10 cc of lymph. Then 3 cc of muscle tissue will form, 2 cc of fat, 1 cc of marrow, and .5 cc of bone. From 1 pound of food, we obtain only .25 cc of semen. If you lose 20 cc of semen in a single ejaculation, you have just spent 60 pounds worth of food and 4 whole pounds of blood. To replace that semen will require that you eat 60 pounds of food (Adhikari 7).

Many athletes and martial artists already know by experience that if they do not engage in sex during a training cycle before a competitive event, they will feel stronger, more courageous, focused, and determined. This is because physical exercise stimulates the upward movement of semen. Therefore, physical exercise is recommended, especially for teenagers and young adults. Medical science supports this.

The Vedas, or Indian books of wisdom, inform us that if one loses semen, or channels it downward, the opposite qualities arise in the heart, such as weakness, cowardice, and a lack of focus.

Interestingly, Dr. David Frawley explains that abstinence from sex is important in disease treatment. It is especially so in the case of mental and nervous disorders because sexual activity increases disturbance and dullness in the mind, thereby reducing mental clarity. We can experience that when abstinence becomes quite natural in acute disease conditions (e.g., fever). It is a way for our body to preserve vitality and use it to combat the disease (192–93).

Furthermore, the ancient Taoists talk about the transformation of wet Yin into dry Yang. Raw semen (Yin) needs to rise to the brain and be transformed into dry Yang. To Taoists, this is the only time when the fullness of Yin/Yang energy transformation comes about. Then, the bones become like steel while remaining as flexible as an infant's. Taoists call this a rejuvenation (Pages 89–95). A serious warrior cannot neglect this point.

As far as Buddhist principles are concerned, human life depends on three elements ("treasures"): a man's semen, the inner energy (*ki*), and mental energy (the power of willingly controlling the mind by obeying the intelligence). If we overexpend any of these, we will die (Szymankiewicz 124).

To conclude, without sexual control, a warrior will never experience his/her full potential. The ability to become strong in body and mind and the ability to control one's sexual energy go hand in hand. Lord Krishna, the Supreme Warrior, tells Arjuna on the battlefield, "I am the strength of the strong, devoid of passion and desire. I am sex life which is not contrary to religious principles, O Arjuna" (Bhagavad Gita 7.11). Lord Krishna links the highest power of a warrior with his ability to spend semen in a controlled manner.

All types of power are diminished when one improperly discharges semen. Great yogis, or mystics, of India emphasize complete continence (sans. *brahmacharya*) as a way to control and channel one's creative energy and, thus, accelerate spiritual progress (Frawley, 193).

Some great examples of classical continence are Greek scientists and philosophers, Pythagoras, Hippocrates, Aristotle, biblical prophets, Elijah, John the Baptist, and Jesus Christ. In more modern times, one may mention Michelangelo, Pascal, Spinoza, Newton, Kant, Beethoven, Thoreau, and many others.

Appendix C

Client testimonials

What people have to say about Ark's training method and approach:

"The journey started on Sunday, 1/7/07, when Ark took me into the gym and said, 'Let's see how strong you are.' Then he did the so-called karate exhaustion plan assessment, which is basically reacting to a whistle and doing push-ups, each time more (starting with one). I got as far as eight whistles—not too good. I started the Transcendental Warrior Achievement Program the next day. Ark has taught me a lot in a short time.

"I know I have a completely new view on how to exercise, when to exercise, and why to exercise. I have increased muscle and reduced body fat. I especially enjoyed the sport-specific strength and endurance work. My son said that my water skiing this season was the best ever. I can honestly say that the time I have spent with Ark has been extremely rewarding. He never gives up on you."

William H.
Age: 55
CPA; Buffalo Grove, Illinois

"As a mother of five children, I truly appreciate the fitness and strength I was able to develop thanks to the warrior program. Ark educates his clients on all aspects of health. I began training with Ark with only some vague goals of losing weight. I actually didn't think having a trainer was necessary. Now, after 6 months, I realize I was mistaken. I have increased strength, cardiovascular endurance, improved appearance, and realized that I am stronger than I previously thought. The right trainer can greatly assist a person in making tremendous fitness strides. Ark takes an interest in his clients' overall well-being—physical, emotional, and spiritual. I would recommend Ark's training approach to anyone who takes a serious, well-rounded approach to health and fitness."

Susan H.
Age: 47
Fabric Artist; Arlington Heights, Illinois

"There came a time in my karate training when I knew that I could not advance anymore without getting physically fit. I then made a decision to get a personal trainer. When I started working with a trainer, my goal was to just get physically fit so I could continue training at an advanced karate level. After I began training with Ark, not only did I lose fat weight, gained strength and stamina, but my goals have evolved to becoming a healthier person psychologically and emotionally.

"Ark is not only about getting you physically trained. The different types of exercises have given me so much self-confidence that is not confined to a gym environment but transfers into all areas of my life. His exercises motivate you to keep working harder and harder to achieve your goals (I love those Crouching Tigers). I really enjoy learning and performing exercises that I never thought I would be able to do. Ark helps you keep track of your eating schedule and maintain a healthy lifestyle. There is never a boring day with Ark at the gym. If you are serious about exercise, health, and becoming the best person you can be, Ark has a plan for you."

Cindy H.
Age: 30
Latin America Operations Coordinator; Round Lake, Illinois

"Hello, let me introduce myself. My name is Ziggy. I was born in Poland, and I am 42 years old. I worked for my local police department's antiterrorist group known as 'Grom (Thunder).' My hobbies included going to the gym, bodybuilding, and martial arts like karate-do and kickboxing. I started my karate and kickboxing practice in Poland as a teenager. Later, due to increased demands at work, I found I did not have time to pursue my combative practice.

"When I came to the USA many years later, I met a personal trainer by the name Ark, who encouraged me to resume my martial arts practice at Xsport gym. He pushed me hard, drawing on my previous experience with karate and kickboxing. Thanks to him, my results were excellent; my body felt stronger and more powerful after his warrior workout. Thus, I started to train with Ark regularly. His methods are professional, and he really knows how to imbue the individual with a true fighting spirit. When you come to work out with Ark, you better be prepared to give 100 percent, because he will expect no less. He puts his whole being into each training session, and I can tell that spirit comes from the bottom of his heart."

Ziggy
Age: 43
Business Owner; Palatine, Illinois

"My exercise goals are to be stronger, more flexible, and create greater balance. Having worked with Ark for only 6 weeks, I already notice that I have better movement. The most enjoyable

aspect of my training is learning proper exercise techniques. I am very fortunate to have met Ark. His knowledge and passion are truly a gift, and my husband and I are blessed."

Zenna Princess Warrior
Age: 51
Office Administrator; Mount Prospect, Illinois

"I am a mother of four children, and it had been several years since I'd worked out regularly. Ark and I started out slowly and gradually increased the difficulty of my exercises. He's recommended a complete program of strength training and cardio training as well as a nutritional plan. I've followed his program consistently and have made steady progress towards my goals. I've gained muscle, lost weight, and increased my overall level of fitness.

"I've had problems with my lower back since I was a teenager. After training with Ark, my back has never been better. The workouts were structured in such a way to put minimal pressure on my lower back while strengthening the muscles in that area. It's made a real difference for me. Ark's enthusiasm for fitness training is contagious. I work out 6–7 days a week now!"

Kimberly D.
Age: 49
Advertising Research; Arlington Heights, Illinois

"When I turned 40, I said to myself, 'I am going to start exercising regularly!' The dusty treadmill and gut were a constant reminder of how that was going. So when a small fitness shop opened nearby, my wife and I did some training sessions and I realized I needed a 'task master' driving me; otherwise, I would never work myself as hard. The storefront operation was short-lived, though, and I had several different trainers with little consistency. They closed, and I was soon back on the couch.

"But when I started with Ark 2 years ago, he provided me a challenge from day one and has ramped it up ever since. He has provided nutritional, physiological, and spiritual guidance all the way. I have lost some weight, but my body fat percentage has gone way down. I definitely am stronger and able to do more for a longer period of time. I don't always ACT on what I have been taught, but Ark doesn't give up!

"I enjoy the variety of his training program. He mixes traditional and nontraditional exercises. We take advantage of the equipment at the club as well as doing some 'low-tech' exercises that are very challenging. Ark has kept changing my program, increasing the difficulty from week to week. He now has me on his 'Transcendental Warrior Achievement Program,' which motivates me even more and makes me responsible for certain monthly goals. I look forward to every session, and I go home SWEATY!"

Andrew V.
Age: 48
Software Developer; Buffalo Grove, Illinois

"In the past, I did not eat lean and healthy and I did not participate in any physical activities. By following Ark's Warrior program of lean diet and good exercise, I was able to achieve and surpass my goals, have tons of energy, and generally feel good about myself and life. Without his program, I don't think my mind would be strong enough to do or come up with this on my own.

Ark and I together implemented a very strict workout program, which included kickboxing. The amount of weight loss was amazing. I lost 73 pounds in just 3 months, mostly body fat. Just to get this weight off the body is a huge relief. Without a doubt, Ark has helped me 100% through this challenge, not just by creating a perfect plan, but also by talking to me and inspiring me as a friend and mentor. There were days when my morale would be low but he always found a way to get my energy and self confidence up in those moments and have me feeling positive for rest of the day.

There is nothing to lose (expect that stubborn weight) and everything to gain (self confidence, newfound love for life and fitness). There is nothing better than looking in the mirror months later and asking yourself, 'Where did the other half of me go?' When people start complimenting you on how good you look and how much weight you lost, that just makes it all worthwhile. To see your family in tears that you were able to accomplish such task and actually get off the path you were on (path to destruction of your health) is just priceless. There is nothing that a strong will and mind cannot achieve in this life."

Arnel V.
Age: 26
Truck driver; Arlington Heights, Illinois

"My goals were to look and feel strong and to be able to compete in strength endurance events. When I first met Ark, I noticed he had a very unique hair style. He gave me a copy of his first book. That's when I realized how much of a freak he was when it came to health and fitness. And he is also all natural, which was very important to me.

"We soon embarked on a journey of physical, mental, and spiritual training that has made me stronger than I could have ever imagined. I found that training is a mental thing as well as physical, and that you can't perform at your best with a bad diet. As for results, I noticed a big difference in my endurance, my strength, my look, and also heart rate recovery. The most enjoyable aspect of training is trying the interesting and different exercises that Ark comes up with. He offers a truly unique program."

Joe Delulio "the Warrior"
Age: 26
Triathlete; Lake Zurich, Illinois

"My goals were to slim down, build muscle, and get healthy mentally and physically. I struggled with my weight, and I joined the gym thinking that I would be able to lose weight on my own. I was wrong.

"When I started working with Ark, I could tell from day one that he was really on the ball and cared about his clients. He designed these challenging routines for me that were fun. He really took time to make up routines that would best help me reach my goals. I enjoyed the variation of routines, and the kickboxing was my favorite. That was the best.

"Ark gave me the encouragement that I could succeed at my weight goals. In addition, to kick off my exercise program, I was given nutritional information on what were the right things to eat. I followed that and got real results. In a year and a half that I worked with Ark, I lost between 35–40 pounds. I could see real definition in my arms, stomach, and legs. I was amazed by the results.

"When I graduated from Ark's warrior program, I had a good idea on how to use a lot of the equipment the proper way and how to change my routines. Having gained so much knowledge on fitness, I could maintain my weight and exercise program on my own. Ark is a wonderful trainer and all-around nice person who cares about you."

Kirsten Calderone
Age: 35
Middle School Science Teacher; Elk Grove Village, Illinois

"In the past, I had a tendency to spend hours in the gym, but never gained the results that I was looking for. Through personal training with Ark, I learned the importance of stretching, diet, and healthy lifestyle habits. I have been training with Ark for approximately 2 months and have noticed increased muscle mass as well as reduction in body fat. I enjoy how the training sessions are broken into different sequences and how we alternate between various workouts.

"Ark is an ally of yours throughout the entire training process. Though his workouts can be intense and grueling, you feel a great sense of accomplishment upon their completion. Ark challenges you to reach your peak performance and is there every step of the way, providing guidance and moral support when exhaustion sets in.

"Not only does he serve as a mentor, but also as a friend. He wants you to succeed, not just for his own benefit, but because he means well and cares deeply about his clients. Ark's popularity among customers within the gym reflects his overall likeability and knowledge as a trainer. In addition, he is physically apt to demonstrate all of the exercises, and his overall level of fitness is astonishing. If you can't see the benefits of doing the warrior challenge program, then you either don't have the work ethic or the desire to attain a higher degree of fitness."

Brian B.
Age: 20
Student; Arlington Heights, Illinois

"I was able to increase muscle mass, strength, and lose excess body fat. The creative types of exercises Ark uses during training sessions keep things interesting. He sets the bar very high for himself and that reflects itself in his client training. Ark expects great results and ensures that clients get in the right frame of mind so that they, too, believe in their ability to achieve those results.

"Ark has a warm, caring approach to his work. His sense of humor helps get you through the really hard work that he is taking you through. It is readily apparent how much he cares about getting the most out of the effort clients put into their training. He checks on their nutrition, sleep, and water intake. He monitors their condition before, during, and after the session, etc. Although Ark takes a very serious and professional approach to his work, he also balances it by keeping a fun, friendly, and enthusiastic tone during all training sessions."

Paul G.
Age: 55
Real Estate Developer; Arlington Heights, Illinois

"Five years ago, I became very ill due to family problems. I was very frail and weak, and I started to have difficulties doing even normal daily activities. My self-esteem was very low, and I was depressed. To deal with all the physical and emotional pain, I was given a myriad of prescriptions. Many of them were addicting and very harmful when taken for long periods of time. I began to feel trapped because the medications were not helping my issues, and I was spending a fortune.

"Then I began a strict workout routine with Ark, and my physical and mental health improved tenfold. I have been able to cut out 90 percent of my prescription drugs. I follow Ark's instructions on nutrition, and I feel energized. He finds a way to motivate and change your mood so you can complete an exciting and vigorous workout. There is communication but also strict discipline.

"Ark helps you to stay focused and positive, which make you succeed in something you never thought you would. Just 1 hour a day of the warrior workout is life changing. Ark is very interested in the well-being of his clients, has compassion on them, and is patient to see them progress. His positive energy is contagious, which makes working out a delightful time."

Blanca M.
Age: 59
Business Owner; Palatine, Illinois

"My experience training with Ark has been exceptional. Ark takes fitness and health to a level that exceeds my expectations! Prior to working with Ark, I felt discontented about my weight and overall health. Finally, I decided to make a lifestyle change. I began to work with Ark about 3 months ago and have never felt better.

"I thought I used to work out and be healthy years ago. As I have learned now, that was not accurate. Ark pushed my limits to a new level, and I see a new horizon ahead of me. I never imagined myself to be this strong and healthy. He has taught me that accomplishing the goal is up to me. And I have never trained that hard!

"Ark also incorporated nutrition into my fitness plan. There were so many misconceptions that I had about what foods were good and bad. He gave me charts and explanations that have helped my eating tremendously. I remember just a few months ago not being able to bend over without struggling. Now I play tennis, jog, and workout on my own. I used to eat horrible and go out to have a few beers. Now I find myself working out and doing positive activities during my free time. Working with Ark is not only about hitting the gym, it's about changing your life!!!"

Maria R.
Age: 28
Student; Chicago, Illinois

"I am a 5-year cancer survivor on a daily chemotherapy that has side effects affecting my daily life. In the past, prior to cancer, exercise and fitness were always an effective tool in maintaining and improving my health. After starting chemotherapy, I joined a fitness facility and wanted to regain health by myself, but after 9 months and still dealing with the side effects of my medications, I felt I would implement a personal trainer.

"Which trainer would I choose? I was interested in someone who would be compassionate about my situation, but most importantly, someone who would be a motivating source. I chose Ark because I saw him in action working with a very challenged client—he was genuinely interested in helping his clients achieve their fitness goals. He watched every rep of exercise, both spotting and offering suggestions to assure their success and safety.

"After working out for less than 6 months, I noticed a dramatic difference in the quality of my life. I successfully conquered the severe fatigue and muscular cramping caused by daily chemotherapy. I feel great emotionally. I still am working on my weight management, but my body feels stronger and is more flexible. Over the last year, I have continued my training with Ark several times per week, never feeling bored with the workouts and always inspired by the enthusiasm he brings to my training session. I feel great and never look back!"

Joyce C.
Age: 58
Project Manager; Arlington Heights, Illinois

"The most important aspect of my fitness journey has been the possibility of developing and acquiring new healthy habits, such as exercising at least four times a week, eating healthy foods at the right time, combining the foods properly, and using good supplements. Ark has become the person who really held me accountable for all of my goals, always willing to give advice, share his knowledge about nutrition, healthy lifestyle habits, etc. He gradually progresses you to

the most challenging exercises, and I enjoy their variety—they help me stay interested and focused. I lost 26 pounds and went down 2 sizes! That is why I feel very lucky to find in Ark a fitness trainer who will lead you to faster results and better performance. Thank you, Ark. Keep it up! You are amazing. God bless you, or Hare Krishna!"

Zulay B.
Age: 47
Sales Manager; Wheeling, Illinois

"I've been trying to shed extra pounds and tone my body since the time I had my son. My results were mediocre and I never achieved what I achieved with Ark in just 8 weeks!! He taught me how important healthy nutrition is and what to eat before and after a strength (or cardio) workout. Most importantly, I learned that to be fit and strong you do not need to eat meat! I love Ark's detailed nutritional plan, which includes my favorite healthy recipes, vitamins, as well as properly selected shake supplements.

Workouts with Ark are different and interesting and often draw the attention of gym members. Once when performing the Krishna Warrior Biceps Curl, I heard a passerby comment, 'Hm, this looks puzzling.' I myself was surprised that you can activate so many muscles with just one exercise! Ark's exercises are amazingly effective and maximize your time at the gym. I see a tremendous difference. I now workout 6 days a week, follow a very healthy vegetarian food regimen, and feel great in my body! Success is not just about harmonizing your physical body but also your mind and soul. I thank God for giving me a chance to know you Ark."

"Your Warrior Kasia"
Age: 28
Massage Therapist; Prospect Heights, Illinois

"When I started working out, I was very intimidated and nervous because I was in terrible shape and had very little knowledge on how to work out properly. My goals were to become healthier, get in a better physical condition, and also to learn more exercises for my goals.

"Ark started me out with a workout that was easy for me to do with confidence, and he gradually increased the levels of difficulty. He is great at putting together workouts and nutritional plans designed for your personal needs that are challenging but not impossible to follow. And he makes the workouts enjoyable to do.

"Ark is very friendly, personable, and a funny guy to talk to. He always gives me positive reinforcement and encouragement, which pushes me forward when I struggle. I am completely comfortable coming to work out on my own now. Ark has equipped me with skills and techniques that I never had. I am in better shape now and have more energy than before thanks to his help."

Lori S.
Age: 46
Homemaker; Arlington Heights, Illinois

"I was at a point in my life where I needed more of a challenge and a focus to get my body toned. I have always been into personal fitness and staying in shape, but I needed something different and more motivating to keep me going and get my body where I wanted it to be. I began working with Ark twice a week about 4 months before my wedding. I absolutely saw a difference in my body and felt a lot healthier and leaner.

"Ark is an amazingly educated and motivating individual that I enjoyed training with and learning from. He helped me to learn how to use a variety of techniques other than the typical weight machines that I was used to using on my own. He encouraged me to try new things by making working out more fun yet challenging each and every time we would meet."

Kim B.
Age: 28
Elementary School Teacher; Buffalo Grove, Illinois

"As a person who is a high-school health teacher and who already works out hard 5–6 days a week, putting on pounds seemed very daunting. I noticed how Ark trained his clients and how much their bodies began to change over time. I decided it was time to get out of my comfort zone and take that challenge.

"The two sessions a week I train with Ark are pretty grueling, making it a 'love/hate' relationship. I love how hard he makes me work, and I know the end of that training hour will be worth it. I learned that any person, regardless of body type or age, can make positive changes, and the focus should be on changing body composition rather than simply losing weight.

"Every 6 weeks, Ark develops a new workout routine. My previous training in the past kept me doing the same exercises over and over. It has been really interesting to see how much stronger I have become. I wasn't even able to do push-ups when I started, and after 8 weeks, I can do sets of them at a time.

"Clothes that I haven't worn in a while are starting to feel loose again. I feel more confident about the way I look because of a more toned appearance. I also have more energy from combining the new fitness routine with a balanced diet.

"I no longer have extreme drops in my blood sugar levels, and mentally, my moods are much 'lighter,' and I can concentrate better.

"I have really enjoyed learning new exercises. Doing the body type quizzes has finally enlightened me on what my real body type is and how I should eat and train to get the best results. As a person who thought I would never need a personal trainer, I would 100 percent recommend Ark's training approach to anyone. I feel proud of myself for taking on the warrior challenge and sticking to it."

Renee D.
Age: 39
High School Health Teacher; Buffalo Grove, Illinois

"My exercise goal is to maintain a high energy level and maintain my weight while getting more muscle tone. I have noticed improvement in all of them. At the age of 60, I am still improving strength and feeling good while learning better ways to exercise and eat. This makes all aspects of life more enjoyable. I realize that I can achieve more. Ark follows his own advice and is a dedicated and 'tough' trainer who makes the journey of improved fitness worthwhile."

Donald C.
Age: 61
Marketing Consultant; Arlington Heights, Illinois

"I planned on going to the gym at least twice a week, but I was struggling. My routines were chosen at random and did not focus on developing any particular part of my body. I was not satisfied with the results, and so I have decided to sign up with Ark. He developed a special set of routines for me so I could tone up and lose weight in a most efficient way. I learned that not only a combination of strength and cardio training will bring results, but that a rigorous nutritional plan and food quality are equally important . . . and I didn't have to wait long for results. Just after a couple of weeks, I have noticed increased energy levels, increased strength, and I dropped a few pounds."

Sebastian L.
Age: 30
Banker; Illinois

"My fitness goal was to tone my whole body, feel stronger, and be happy. After doing Ark's workout, I feel energized and my bodily pains go away. Of course, to get full benefits from the workouts, one must follow Ark's practical nutritional suggestions, which are so helpful, along with the whole monitoring process he implements. To me, communication and sharing the training experience is as important as the workout itself, and that's what I get from the workout of my life."

Ana R.
Age: 45
Hair Stylist; Buffalo Grove, Illinois

"Ark pushed me to work very hard while always watching my technique to make sure I was working out safely. Education in proper techniques was very important to avoid injury. Two years ago, I was fat and out of shape. Now, I look at my very much improved physique and am thankful that I decided to work out with Ark. All of the hard work has paid off! I even get comments from strangers about my toned body."

Vicki R.
Age: 50
Swimming Coach; Buffalo Grove, Illinois

"We met Ark at Xsport, and he, my husband, and I just hit if off. He told us up front we will reach our goal, but we will have to work hard. When we start our sessions with Ark, we are warriors. He truly cares about us and is very determined we reach our fitness goal. He takes time to listen to our individual fitness concerns. We were able to change old eating habits and are trying alternative foods that we otherwise wouldn't have tried were we not with Ark. I [Kurt] have more muscle tone, strength, flexibility. Says Lisa: 'It feels great to make progress (my pants fit better) but also to know there's more growth and challenges ahead.'"

Kurt and Lisa B.
Ages: 38 and 37
Store Manager and Customer Service; Buffalo Grove, Illinois

"I had a hard time making it through a long day at work, and then I met someone who was training with Ark. In the beginning, we were about the same speed and then it became more difficult to keep up with him. I asked him what he was doing to have as much energy throughout the day, and he introduced me to Ark.

"I have been training with Ark for 9 months now, and my goals include overall physical wellness. The two aspects of training that I've enjoyed the most would be the challenge of the Transcendental Warrior Achievement Program, which means meeting the goals set each month, and kickboxing, which works all the muscles in the body. Since training with Ark, I feel full of energy throughout the day, and I can get my job done even better. Ark has the knowledge to increase your physical fitness and ability to motivate."

Jason L.
Age: 32
Store Manager; Lake Zurich, Illinois

"Training Ark's way is a great way to make commitment to yourself, which is not always easy. It is not enough for him to give you advice on how to exercise right to make all the muscles work the way they are supposed. He also helps you implement a healthy lifestyle change. And your hard work and persistency will pay off in the long run.

"If you have a goal that you want to accomplish and you follow the plan set for you, the results will be yours. As for me, the fitness goals included high-energy living, looking and feeling great, and, of course, toning. I have lost about 10 pounds of body fat and gained 3 pounds of muscle in the 3 months of my training with Ark. I exercise 5–6 times a week and really like the way I look and feel. After the workout, I feel full of energy for the whole day. I am very proud of myself to accomplish this, and without Ark's help, it would have never happened. He is a great person to work with."

Renata T.
Age: 33
Insurance Company President; Buffalo Grove, Illinois

"I started out 10 months ago and my fitness goals included a better understanding of what I need to do to maintain health and fitness level. At first, I had results pretty quickly, but after a few months into it, I had hit a plateau and didn't see any increase in muscle or loss of weight.

"After reassessing my nutrition, we decided to increase the daily amount of protein. That helped, and I began seeing results again. Education about nutrition was definitely an important part of my training because without knowing how to eat right, I wouldn't be able to reach the level I'm at right now. Plus, Ark always has new and different exercises to challenge me with, and I've enjoyed learning them."

James A.
Age: 37
QA Engineer; Bensenville, Illinois

"I started with Ark three times a week. We do strength training twice a week and kickboxing once a week. I really enjoy kickboxing. My goals revolve around losing weight and getting into shape.

"I have struggled with my weight most of my life, and in the last several years, my weight has really jumped and yo-yoed. I decided I needed someone to motivate me since I always had an excuse not to exercise. I hate every minute of it, but I love how I feel after the workout is over. Well, actually, after the pain subsides.

"I like having more energy and sleeping better at night. My clothes fit better as well. Ark also tries to give me some guidance on nutrition, but I am bad at following it. I've always been a meat/potatoes girl, so changing my diet and lifestyle has been very difficult. I haven't achieved all my fitness goals, but generally when I do work with Ark on a consistent basis, I usually have more energy and I feel stronger. The journey is usually very painful and very difficult, but I like Ark's spirit and the way he tries to motivate his clients. He never gives up, and he really pushes you further than you can push yourself."

Rebecca L.
Age: 37
Senior Principal Systems Engineer; Lake Zurich, Illinois

"I feel my exercise program helped me to be healthier physically and emotionally. I noticed a more toned body and stronger muscles. My cardio endurance improved. I reduced my stress level and built confidence.

"Ark is very encouraging and easy to work with but pushes me to do my personal best. He explained to me the importance of focusing during training, as well as gave specific feedback with each exercise.

"My current diet was recorded and examined by Ark, after which I received specific recommendations from him. He also gave me several articles on healthier eating and shared some

good nutritional Web sites. Ark is very precise in his approach to training and will provide you with a complete plan."

Mary S.
Age: 53
Middle School Teacher; Arlington Heights, Illinois

"Ark puts his warrior candidates through a 1-hour fitness assessment in order to tailor a training program to reach their specific goals. We discussed nutritional habits, workout experience, and he measured my current physical condition.

"In addition to exercising on my own, I met with Ark once a week and trained with low weight/high repetitions to build core strength, increase agility, and improve overall endurance and power. Along the way, my progressively harder workouts were maximized by changes in my diet that he had recommended. The sessions were strenuous. However, the mental discipline instilled by Ark will get you through. In 10 weeks, I lost 4 percent body fat and gained 3 pounds of lean body mass."

Vince N.
Age: 46
Actor; Long Grove, Illinois

"Fitness should be part of our daily routine. Keeping your body in shape and healthy really makes you change your lifestyle. One of the by-products of such a healthy lifestyle is that our productivity increases day by day.

"As for myself, I definitely lowered my body fat level and have increased energy levels. I especially enjoyed working my lower body.

"During the course of my training with Ark, I realized that having the right nutrition is one of the important factors in getting healthy and fit. If you want to be more efficient in your workout, have a specific goal and be more motivated about it. Work with Ark."

Richard N.
Age: 25
Aspiring Golfer, Photographer; Palatine, Illinois

"I have been exercising consistently my entire adult life. But at age 46, my body was not responding as I wished, despite spending 5–6 days per week at the gym. Ark assessed my fitness level and body fat and with careful consideration, tailored 10 weeks of individualized workouts for me. Each session left me physically exhausted yet exhilarated! Workouts changed from session to session and were always challenging and stimulating and gave me new ideas for workouts on my own. Equally important, Ark corrected my eating habits, and I easily fell into several new

eating patterns and commitments. In 10 weeks, I lost 15 pounds and lowered my body fat by 5 percent.

Dyanne W.
Age: 48
Librarian; Arlington Heights, Illinois

"The most enjoyable aspect of training is its challenge. Ark personally determines the unique workouts for me every 6 weeks. He has a sincere desire and commitment to me in the matter of improving my health. Since I have begun training with Ark, I feel more energy and I look better. I would recommend Ark's warrior workout challenge because he walks his talk. I respect Ark for that."

Nirel K.
Age: 37
Vice President; Buffalo Grove, Illinois

"I have been going to the gym and training with Ark for over a year and love every minute of it. I enjoy the variety that he has to offer in regards to his knowledge of different ways of training. I love knowing that when I go into the gym, it's not going to be just lifting or just cardio. It could be either or none or we may do kickboxing instead.

"My fitness goals always change with the seasons, but, above all, my goal is to keep myself in good physical condition and healthy. The results I have noticed have run a broad spectrum from just straight weight loss to the building of my endurance to be able to run and compete in triathlons.

"A key result of working out with a trainer and being in shape is the ability of your body to sustain itself and not get tired throughout the day. I am grateful for having a trainer who is willing to push me and not settle for anything less than the best. Ark is a strong trainer and is on top of his game."

Zach N.
Age: 28
IT; Arlington Heights, Illinois

"My friends recommended Ark as an excellent personal trainer. I never before worked with a personal trainer, so I didn't know what to expect. My sessions with Ark exceeded my expectations, in large part because his preparation, professionalism, and passion for fitness is exceptional. Even though I started training with him only recently, the quality of his instruction persuaded me to sign up for additional sessions. His training approach is very thorough,

consisting of a dietary plan, numerous exercises, and the motivation to push myself with every workout toward a higher level of performance."

Elzbieta S.
Age: 53
Quality Assurance Lab Technician; Buffalo Grove, Illinois

"I am 50 years old, and thanks to Ark, I feel many years younger. Ark is very helpful in making your training experience a great one. Ark provides many insights into how I can improve the quality of my life and my overall fitness. I have been training for 3 years now and would definitely recommend this program to anyone who is serious about improving their physical and mental outlook."

Rodolfo O.
Age: 51
Insurance Agent; Arlington Heights, Illinois

"When I joined Xsport Fitness, I wanted to develop a healthy style of living and feel better. I also wanted to fight my own laziness and lack of motivation to work hard. Ark's holistic approach to training sounded engaging and promising to me. His routine, in combination with his eating plan, brought my weight down by about 10 pounds in 2½ months. My body fat dropped from 33 percent to 27 percent. I was mostly surprised by the changes in the way my body looked. Ark targeted exactly what needed to be improved. He clearly knows what he is doing and delivers results. I feel healthier, younger, and more feminine. I am proud of my accomplishments.

"Ark's warrior style of personal training (for which I was not prepared at all) and his personal qualities makes me believe I am being guided by a knowledgeable athlete and a determined coach who makes me sweat and laugh at the same time. Whenever I am just about to give up, his warrior attitude and great jokes uplift me and spur me on. In addition, he approaches his job from a spiritual viewpoint, all while putting a dash of fun into the practice.

"Thank you, Ark! I guess I do 'feel the power,' as you like to encourage your clients. The power of a mind over a body."

Yelena K.
Age: 40
Elementary School Teacher; Wheeling, Illinois

GALLERY

Here are some of recently taken pictures that I decided to include. I had just then completed my 3 months of intense hypertrophy mesocycles that resulted in an increase of at least 6 pounds of lean body mass. I ended up weighing 162 pounds with approximately 7 percent body fat. My normal weight fluctuates between 152 and 154 with a body fat (BF) percentage between 7 and 8. During martial arts training cycles which focus on power anaerobic endurance drills and technique, I maintain a slightly lighter weight (150–152 pounds) with lower BF percentage (5–6).

My nutritional plan for increasing muscle was consuming at least 200 grams of protein daily (mostly from whey protein, raw milk, and cheese), with monthly increases (up to 250 grams), with at least 25 percent of healthy fats (such as almonds, nuts, raw milk, and cheese).

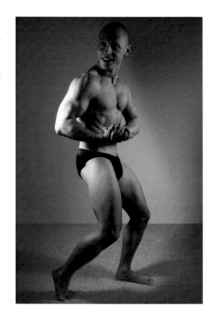

My calorie intake increased from my usual 3,000 to around 4,000 a day, which gave me a fat/protein/carbohydrate ratio 25 percent fat/25 percent protein/50 percent carbohydrates.

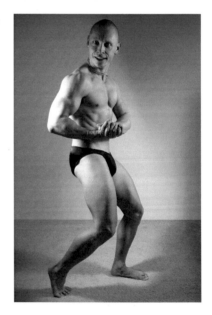

The focus was on medium-tempo movements with heavier weights of around 85 percent of one round maximum (1RM).

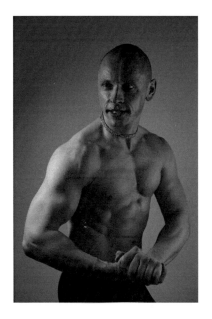

Most of my gains came in the upper body and that was my focus in the 3-month hypertrophy cycle.

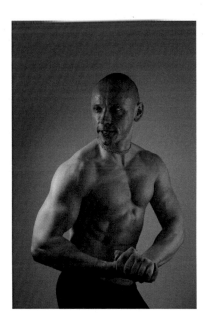

I never deprive myself of healthy vegetable carbohydrates in order to feel good and strong during my workout and throughout the day. My fruit consumption is lower.

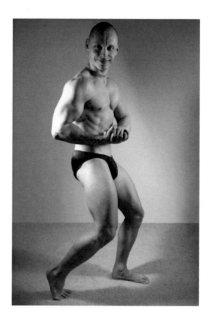

My preferred leg exercises are One-legged Squats, Up-and-Down Lunges, and Olympic Squats. I avoid leg extension machines.

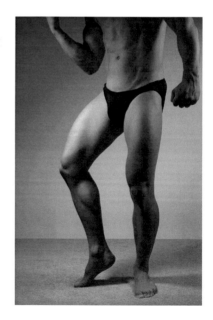

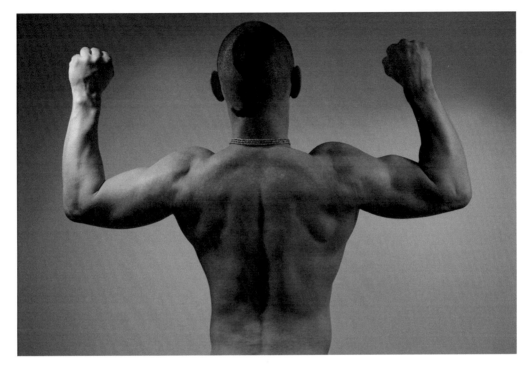

In karate, there are some great exercises for the lower back, such as punching on your stomach. A strong back means you can bench-press more weight and punch or push harder.

Bent over Rows and Pull-ups are my favorite back exercises.

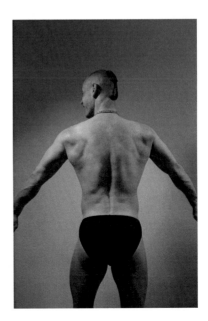

In martial arts, it is important to balance your upper body musculature with core and leg muscles.

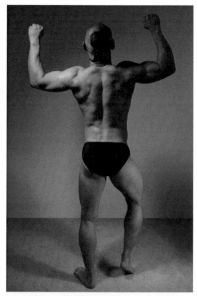

This is the "Thanks to Krishna" pose.

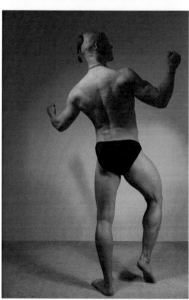

This is the "Krishna Power" pose.

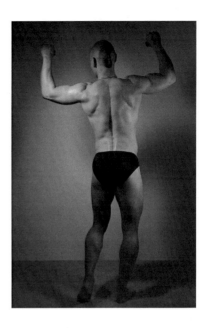

Another "Krishna Power" pose.

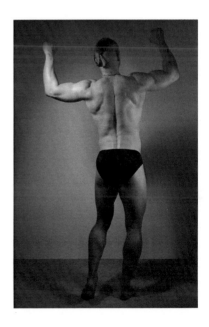

Back and shoulder development are crucial to martial arts such as karate.

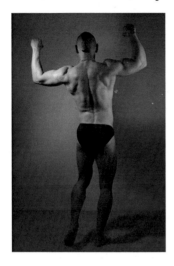 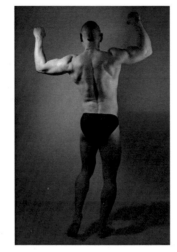 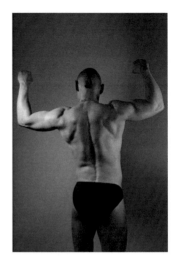

It's hard to stay serious sometimes.

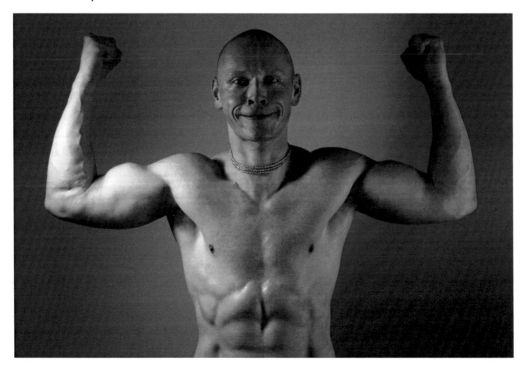

I think I will give up.

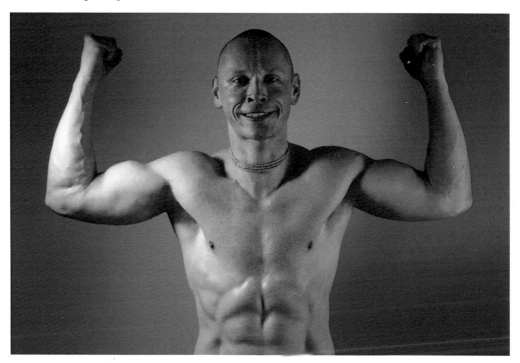

Couldn't hold it anymore! *Hare Krishna!*

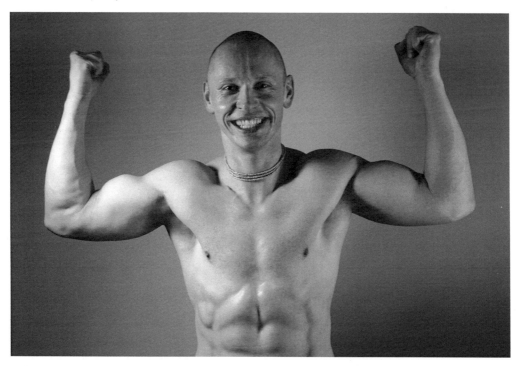

Is it finally over now, Rich?

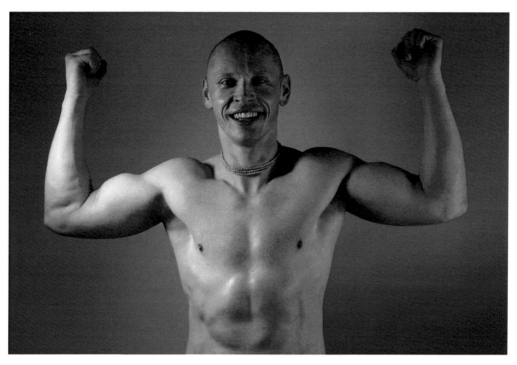

Okay, I am a little tired of this high time under tension.

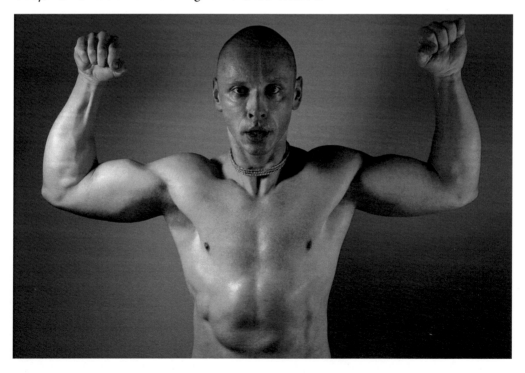

Should I still hold them up?

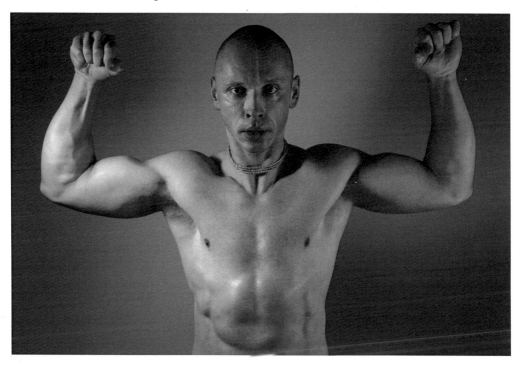

I can still do it for Krishna if I need to . . .

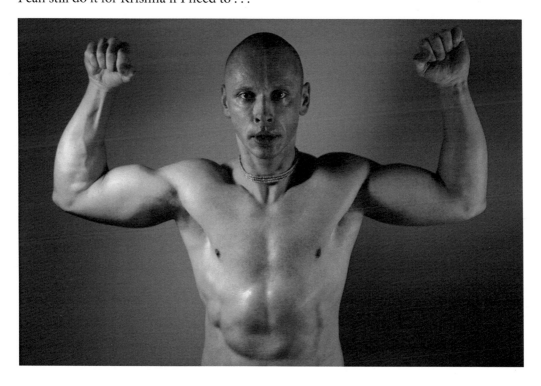

All right, I really need some ninja juice now.

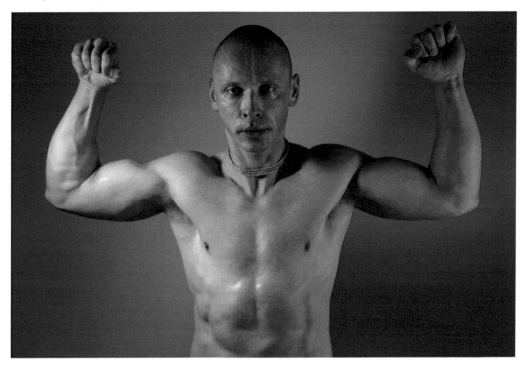

Are you really serious about what you're doing?

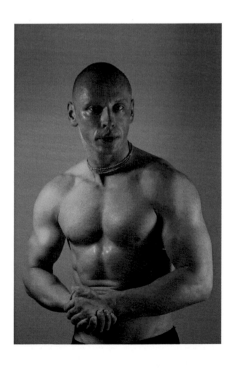

Sometimes I wonder if I am really doing this for Krishna or for my own self. Maybe I am partial?

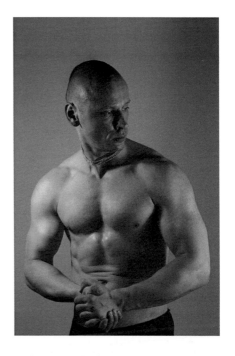

Krishna tells Arjuna, the great warrior, that he is not this body but a spirit soul within. And yet we have to work with this body for the whole time of our material sojourn.

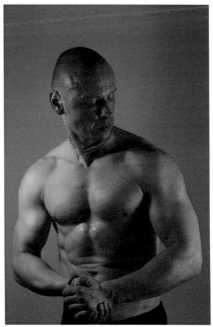

Is Rich finally done shooting these pictures? I just want to go home, eat some *prasadam* (holy food), and listen to Hare Krishna music.

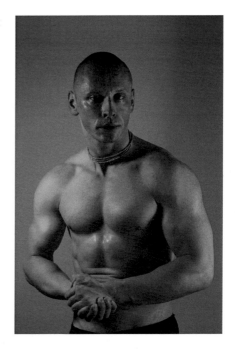

Focus on the mission! (This is for you, Jerry. Thanks for your loud Krishna chants.)

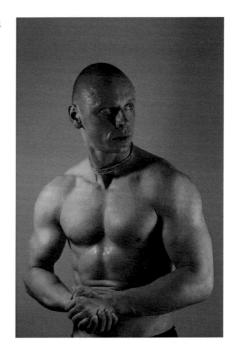

Core development (abdominals, oblique muscles, as well as lower back) lies at the basis of martial arts and many sports.

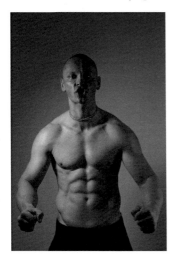 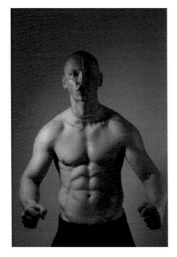 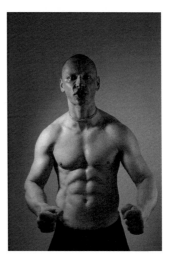

I've had a strong inclination toward martial arts since my childhood.

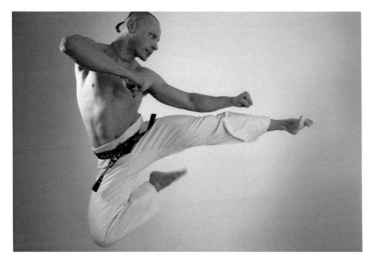

Still a little crazy about it now.

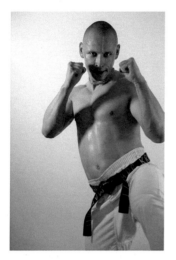
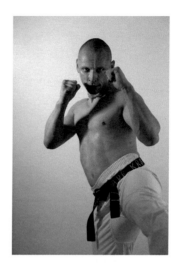

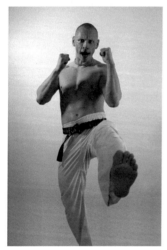
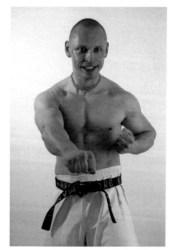

GLOSSARY

Warrior Names that you can adopt with the addition of *DAS* (servant) during the course of your training.

Abhimanyu: This powerful warrior is the son of Arjuna. He is said to be an incarnation of the moon demigod's son. He fought with extreme bravery in the great Battle of Kurukshetra 5,000 years ago and left his body there.

Arjuna: This universally famous warrior, the best archer in the world, is the son of rain demigod Indra. He is known as Krishna's dear friend, and he heard *Bhagavad-Gita* (the Song of God) from Lord Krishna on the battlefield of Kurukshetra 5,000 years ago. The name *Arjuna* means "one of pure deeds." Arjuna is said to be an incarnation of the ancient sage Nara.

Asvatthama: This warrior is the son of the great martial teacher Dronacarya. He is said to be a partial incarnation of Shiva, the god of destruction.

Balarama: Lord Krishna's eternal brother who sometimes appears in the material world to enact pastimes. He is no different from the Lord himself.

Bhima: Sired by Vayu, the wind demigod, Bhima, is Arjuna's famous brother, known for his immense strength and skill in fighting with a mace. After the Battle of Kurukshetra, he was installed by King Yudhisthira as crown prince.

Bhishmadeva: Known as the grandfather of the fighters. After the Battle of Kurukshetra, Bhishmadeva gave instructions on religion and morality while lying on the bed of arrows.

Dhrstaketu: A great warrior who befriended the brothers Arjuna, Bhima, Yudhisthira, Nakula, and Sahadeva. He supplied them with a huge division of soldiers for the Kurukshetra war. He left his body on the battlefield. He is said to be an incarnation of one of the celestial beings (Vishvadevas).

Garuda: Bird carrier of Lord Vishnu (incarnation of Krishna who is in charge of maintenance of the universe).

Ghototkacha: This is Bhima's son, who was a leader of Rakshasas (monsters possessing mystic powers). Ghatotkacha assisted Arjuna and his brothers in the war. He left his body on the battlefield.

Hanuman: The famous monkey warrior sired by the wind demigod Vayu, who is known as the perfect servant of Lord Rama (Krishna's incarnation in a previous age known as "the perfect ruler") and who assisted Lord Rama in regaining his kingdom and wife.

Krishna: Said by the Vedas to be God, the Supreme Person, who is the origin of all incarnations of the Godhead, such as Vishnu, Rama, Narasimha, etc. Before the grand Battle of Kurukshetra, Krishna spoke the *Bhagavad-Gita*, or moral instructions, to Arjuna and the other assembled warriors.

Nakula: Arjuna's brother, who was renowned for his expertise with a sword. He was sired by the Ashvini demigods. He was a *maharatha* warrior, or one who could fight with a thousand soldiers at once.

Narasimha Deva: Half-man, half-lion incarnation of Krishna, who descended to the material world to protect His devoted servant Prahlada. Narasimha removes all obstacles from the spiritual path of His devotee.

Parasurama: A sage said to be an empowered incarnation of Vishnu (Krishna). Millions of years ago, he annihilated all the warriors of the world after his father, Jamadagni, had been killed by a king named Kartavirya. Parasurama is an expert in the Vedic military arts. He was the martial teacher of Bhishma, Drona, Karna, and many other great fighters.

Rakshasa: A powerful, ugly-looking monster that possesses not only physical strength but also mystical power such as the ability to change appearance.

Sahadeva: The youngest brother of Arjuna, fathered by the Ashvini demigods. He is famous for his perceptive powers and intelligence. He was appointed as King Yudhisthira's personal advisor after the Kurukshetra battle.

Shiva: The demigod who is responsible for the annihilation of the material cosmos.

Vishnu: The Supreme Lord's expansion in certain parts of the spiritual sky and also for the creation and maintenance of the material universe. When Vishnu descends to the material world, He is known for fighting and destroying many demons.

Yaksha: Ghostly followers of Kuvera, the treasurer demigod.

Yudhisthira: The eldest brother of the five Pandavas (others are Arjuna, Bhima, Nakula, Sahadeva) sired by the demigod of religion (Dharma). He performed a Rajasuya sacrifice which established him as world emperor. Yudhisthira is most famous for his adherence to virtue and truth and is also known as Ajatashatru, or "one who has no enemies." After the Kurukshetra war, he ruled for 36 years.

BIBLIOGRAPHY

Adhikari, Navayauvana Dasa. *Lessons from the Ayurveda.* USA: New Jaipur Press, 1978.

Chernack, Doug. *Men's Fitness: Unilateral Training: Build Balanced Muscle with This Specialized, One-Sided Workout Strategy.* Smart Training. Weider Publications, 2002; Gale Group, 2002.

Danavir, Swami. *Brain Gain, The Wisdom of Celibacy and Chastity.* Kansas City, MO: Rupanuga Vedic College, 2005.

Dharma, Krishna. *Mahabharata: The Greatest Spiritual Epic of All Time.* Los Angeles, USA: Torchlight Publishing, 1999.

EatSolar.com

Essential Science Publishing. *Essential Oils Desk Reference.* USA: ESP, 2007.

"Foods with High Purine." 2007. Kosmix Corporation. www.right health.com. Online.

Frawley, David. *Ayurvedic Healing. A Comprehensive Guide.* 1989. Delhi, India: Motilal Banarsidass Publishers, 1995.

G., Zach. "Training for the Endomorph." Bodybuilding.com. September 10, 2002.

Gamboa, Patrick. Consultation conducted on June 11, 2007, through International Sports Sciences Association's Question Board.

Gastelu, Daniel, and Frederick Hatfield. *Specialist in Performance Nutrition. The Complete Guide.* 1995. Carpinteria, California: The International Sports Sciences Association, 2000.

Harting, Marcella V., and G. I. "Atom" Bergstrom. *Yes, No, Maybe Chronobiotic Nutrition.* Paradise Valley, Arizona: Yes, No, Maybe Publishing, 2004.

(1) Hatfield, Frederick C., ed. *Fitness: The Complete Guide.* 1992. Santa Barbara, California: The International Sports Sciences Association, 1996.

(2) Hatfield, Frederick C., ed. *Fitness: The Complete Guide.* 1992. Santa Barbara, California: The International Sports Sciences Association, 2004.

ISSA. "Sculpt That Body: Train for Your Body Type!" Bodybuilding.com. June 27, 2003.

Krishnapada, Swami. *Spiritual Warrior III, Solace for the Heart in Difficult Times.* Washington, D.C.: Hari-Nama Press, 2000.

Lad, Vasant. *The Complete Book of Ayurvedic Home Remedies.* New York, New York: Harmony Books, 1998.

Mercola, Joseph. *Dr. Mercola's Total Health Program.* Schaumburg, Illinois: Mercola.com, 2005.

Munn, et al. "Contralateral effects of unilateral resistance training: a meta-analysis." *Journal of Applied Physiology*, November 25, 2003.

Page, Michael. *The Power of Ch'I: An Introduction to Chinese Mysticism and Philosophy.* San Francisco, California: Thorsons, 1988.

Pearl, Bill, ed., and Leroy R. Perry Jr., D.C., ed. *Bill Pearl's Key to the Inner Universe: Encyclopedia on Weight Training.* 1982. Phoenix, Oregon: Bill Pearl Enterprises Inc. Physical Fitness Architects, 2000.

Pearl, Bill. "The Vegetarian Bodybuilder." http://ksteveh.tripod.com/pearl.html.

(1) Prabhupada, A. C. Bhaktivedanta Swami. *Bhagavad-Gita As It Is.* 1983. Victoria, Australia: The Bhaktivedanta Book Trust, 1994.

(2) Prabhupada, A. C. Bhaktivedanta Swami. 9 vols. *Sri Chaitanya-Caritamrita.* Australia: The Bhaktivedanta Book Trust, 1996.

(3) Prabhupada, A. C. Bhaktivedanta Swami. 18 vols. *Shrimad Bhagavatam.* USA: The Bhaktivedanta Book Trust, 1987.

(4) Prabhupada, A .C. Bhaktivedanta Swami. *The Higher Taste.* USA: The Bhaktivedanta Book Trust, 1991.

(5) Prabhupada, A. C. Bhaktivedanta Swami. *The Journey of Self-Discovery.* USA: The Bhaktivedanta Book Trust, 1990.

(6) Prabhupada, A. C. Bhaktivedanta Swami. *The Nectar of Devotion: The Complete Science of Bhakti Yoga.* 1970. Australia: The Bhaktivedanta Book Trust, 1982.

(7) Prabhupada, A. C. Bhaktivedanta Swami. *The Science of Self-Realization.* Australia: The Bhaktivedanta Book Trust, 1997.

Rosen, Steven. *Diet for Transcendence.* 1987. *Food for the Spirit.* Torchlight Publishing, Inc: USA, 1997.

Saag, K. G., and H. Choi. "Epidemiology, risk factors, and lifestyle modifications for gout." *Arthritis Res. Ther.* 8 Suppl 1: S2. doi: 10.1186/ar1907. PMID 16820041, 2006.

Sheldon, William H., S. S. Stevens, et al. *The Varieties of Human Physique: An Introduction to Constitutional Psychology*. New York and London: Harper & Brothers Publishers, 1940.

Staley, Charles. *Special Topics in Martial Arts Conditioning*. USA: Myo-Dynamics Publication, 1996.

Szymankiewicz, Janusz, and Jaromir Sniegowski. *Kung Fu/Wu Shu*. Szczecin: Wydawnictwo "Glob," 1987.

Tiwari, Maya. *A Life of Balance. The Complete Guide to Ayurvedic Nutrition & Body Types with Recipes*. Rochester, Vermont: Healing Arts Press, 1995.

Tsatsouline, Pavel. *The Naked Warrior*. St. Paul, MN: Dragon Door Publications, Inc., 2004.

(1) Underhill, Nathan. "Training for the Ectomorph." Teenbodybuilding.com. March 7, 2002.

(2) Underhill, Nathan. "Training for the Mesomorph." Teenbodybuilding.com. March 7, 2002.

Vikasa, Bhakti Swami. *A Beginner's Guide to Krishna Consciousness*. India: Bhakti Vikasa Swami, 1994.

Watson, George. *Nutrition and Your Mind. The Psychochemical Response*. New York: Harper & Row Publishers, 1972.

Weis, Dennis. "Bill Pearl's Super Nutrition Seminar." Bodybuilding.com.

Whitley, David. "Peripheral Heart Action." NaturalStrength.com, October 7, 2006.

Wolcott, William L., and Trish Fahey. *The Metabolic Typing Diet*. USA: Doubleday, a Division of Random House, Inc., 2000.

Yessis, Michael. *Kinesiology of Exercise*. Lincolnwood, Illinois: Masters Press, 1992.

INDEX

ENDNOTES

1. The preliminary cleansing phase recommended in the book is not a substitute for a complete cleansing regimen, such as Stanley Burroughs' Master Cleanse, the liver, or colon cleanse. It merely helps to relieve the digestive system of the unnecessary workload we overburden it with, thus helping the body in functioning at its optimal level. Complete cleansing should never be done during periods of intense physical work, such as sports training, fitness training, or even moderate-intensity strength training.

2. Research demonstrates that lemon essential oil promotes clarity and invigorates. It is highly antiseptic and antitumoral. It reduces acidity in the body, thus aiding in breaking down and releasing toxins from your body (ESP 72–73).

3. The physical structure (movements) of this meditation comes from Kyokushin karate, and the internal structure (thoughts, visualizations, vibrations) from bhakti-yoga, or yoga of love.

4. This *ki (prana)* then becomes transformed from subtle material life air to purified spiritual energy, far more potent than subtle *ki*. Whatever is not used in conscious connection with the Supreme Warrior becomes material and binding to the material world. Connect with Krishna through Yoga.

5. Obtain only a high therapeutic-grade essential oil and not a mere imitation oil that smells good. Peppermint oil's fragrant influence is purifying and stimulating to the mind, and as we know, the mind is directly connected to the body (ESP 89).

6. For some people with back problems, only rounding the back (flexing) causes back pain, and for others, arching (extending) will create pain. The exercise modification included here is for persons who have an extension bias.

7. Same as 6.

8. For some people with back problems, only rounding the back (flexing) causes back pain, and for others, arching (extending) will create pain. The exercise modification included here is for persons who have a flexion bias.

9. For the purpose of limiting the volume of the book, I chose not to describe and illustrate stretching exercises.

10. As a side note, it is important to mention that a typical martial arts punch (e.g., karate) starts with the twist of the feet, hips, and then the torque of the upper body. The torque of the upper body, starting with the oblique muscles and rectus abdominis, is where your punch can gain more power by strength and acceleration combined. The Tiger Push-up will be so helpful because it puts a great amount of stress on the abdominal area.

11. Same as 6.

12. Same as 6.

13. Same as 6.

14. Starting strength is defined as the number of muscles fibers recruited for work at once, or in the shortest time possible.

15. Descend phase occurs at the beginning of any movement, for instance, rearing back to throw a ball.

16. Amortization occurs when you change from moving backward to a forward move. This is also called static strength.

17. There still is a controversy on whether one can work a certain portion of a muscle, or is it just one single muscle contracting as one unit. This newer hypothesis propounds that it does not matter whether one does Crunches or leg lifts (to target upper or lower abs); they still work the same muscle. Nor does it matter whether one works a muscle at a certain angle of movement. It is still a single muscle, and its shape will depend on one's genetics. One can only increase or decrease the muscle size, just like one can inflate or deflate a balloon.

18. New evidence suggests that holding one's breath during the rising up portion of a sit-up or any kind of physical (concentric) exertion, for that matter, creates more muscular strength, as well as intra-abdominal pressure to stabilize the spine (Yessis 65). A beginner (i.e., a deconditioned individual) or a person with high blood pressure should not hold their breath during the concentric portion of any exercise, as this may cause undue changes in the blood pressure and cause internal trauma or fainting. Proper instruction on breathing is a must for beginners and persons with medical conditions.

19. Same as 6.

20. A typical martial arts punch (e.g., karate) starts with the twist of the feet, hips, and then the torque of the upper body. The torque of the upper body, starting with the oblique muscles and rectus abdominis, is where your punch can gain more power by strength and acceleration combined. The Reverse Tiger Push-up will be so helpful because it puts a great amount of stress on the abdominal area.

21. Same as 6.

22. There are three types of muscle fibers in skeletal muscle. Each muscle has a mixture of fast, medium, and slow twitch fibers. Fast twitch fibers should be trained, especially by power athletes; medium twitch by those who want to increase muscle size; and slow twitch by those who want to increase muscle endurance and not necessarily size or strength.

23. Same as 6.

24. Same as 6.

25. Somatype of the individual means "the patterning of the morphological components, as expressed by the three numerals (Sheldon 7)." The first numeral indicates endomorphic body type; the second numeral, mesomorphic body type; and the last numeral indicates an ectomorph. For example, if a person is a pure ectomorph, his or her body type number would be 117. If he/she is an equal mix of mesomorph and endomorph, with a small amount of ectomorphy, the number would be something like 661.

26. The other seven, being autonomic, carbo-oxidative, electrolyte/fluid balance, acid/alkaline balance, endocrine type, blood type, and prostaglandin balance.

27. Some questions were omitted, and many were paraphrased. I also broke down Pita, Vata, and Kapha into their respective universal elements (water, ether, earth, etc.).

28. A rating system that indicates the different speed with which carbohydrates are processed into glucose (a simple sugar in the bloodstream used as the major energy source) by the body.

29. William Wolcott used George Watson's findings to refine his own system of metabolic typing.

30. A. C. Bhaktivedanta Swami Prabhupada, the founder of the International Society for Krishna Consciousness.

31. When one chants 3,000 names of Vishnu, the effect will be equal to the chanting of one name of Krishna (Srimad Bhagavatam 1.19.6 purport).

32. You may, however, chant everywhere, even without your beads. The sound vibration has descended directly from the spiritual world and cannot be touched by the material energy.

33. Same as 6.

34. Same as 6.

35. Same as 6.

36. Same as 6.

37. Same as 6.

38. Same as 6.

39. Same as 8.

40. Some fitness experts agree that muscles in the body are connected through some soft or subtle software, and contracting, for example, your gluteus maximus (buttock), will generate more force in the neighboring muscles such as the thighs (Tsatsouline 35–72). This can, perhaps, be explained on the basis of neural firings in the muscle tissues.

41. Same as 6.

42. Same as 6.

43. Same as 6.

44. Same as 6.

45. Same as 6.

46. A synthetic hormone that increases the chance of contracting cancer.

47. It should also be known that Bill stopped using steroids by 1961 and had before used them only for short periods under a doctor's supervision.

48. This commandment is interpreted by people as only applying to murder of another human being.

49. The analog of semen in women is the fluid of vaginal lubrications, which is even more precious than male semen because women's weaker nerves make the loss of the female seed more dangerous than the male's (Danavir 52).

ABOUT THE AUTHOR

Arkadiusz (Ark) Madej, an International Sports Sciences Association certified fitness trainer, specialist in performance nutrition, fitness therapy, and martial arts conditioning, has been an avid practitioner of Kyokushin karate since the age of 13. He currently works as a personal trainer at Xsport Fitness in Arlington Heights, Illinois. Visit him at www.Krishnawarriors.com.

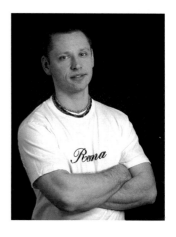

As a boy, Ark was fascinated by powerful warriors and wanted to take karate lessons. Being a spiritually oriented child, he promised the Lord that when he could practice martial arts, he would strive to become the best he could for the Lord's sake. Shortly after that, Arkadiusz happily attended his first martial arts class.

During the course of his karate practice, Arkadiusz developed an interest in learning how to conquer the mind. He knew that the great masters of past ages praised mental strength as necessary to combative advancement. He was also convinced that as a warrior of the Lord, he must control his passions and overcome his weaknesses. He set high standards for himself, but nothing seemed effective. Despite reading many books on Zen and applying what he could, Arkadiusz realized that amid many vague and unattractive descriptions of Zen perfection, and merely by his own strength, he could not subdue his mind and senses. He knew that without this power, he would not be able to be a good warrior or a genuine servant of the Supreme.

During a midnight workout in 1997, he cried out to the Lord to teach him real Zen. Otherwise, he felt helpless to fulfill his promise of becoming a great warrior. He told the Lord that whether he awarded him real knowledge or not, he would never give up his determination to control his mind according to the promise he had made as a boy.

Before long, when he was in college, he met a disciple of A. C. Bhaktivedanta Swami Prabhupada. This disciple's name was Candramauli Swami. The swami and two of his assistants had come to town to present *Bhagavad-gita As It Is*, in accordance with Master Orayen's order that all disciples preach Krishna consciousness.

Seeing great warriors on the cover of the book presented by the visitors, Arkadiusz immediately wanted to read it to see if it could help him fulfill his promise to the Lord. To his delight, in reading the *Bhagavad-gita*, he found that the Supreme Lord spoke to a perplexed warrior on the battlefield, who experienced difficulty controlling his mind and serving the Lord favorably.

In the course of time, as Arkadiusz deepened his studies and realizations of the *Bhagavad-Gita,* he published the Transcendental Warrior book series for spiritual warriors, which fully delineates the science of conquering the mind and becoming the best human being you can be. These books can be obtained at Krishnawarriors.com. The book you are holding in your hand, *Krishna Warrior Fitness Challenge,* is a manual for becoming functionally strong, primarily in body but also in mind.